Advanced Topics of Computed Tomography

Advanced Topics of Computed Tomography

Edited by **Marcus Lewis**

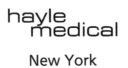

New York

Published by Hayle Medical,
30 West, 37th Street, Suite 612,
New York, NY 10018, USA
www.haylemedical.com

Advanced Topics of Computed Tomography
Edited by Marcus Lewis

International Standard Book Number: 978-1-63241-022-1 (Hardback)

Printed in the United States of America.

Contents

Preface

This book offers in-depth description on advanced topics in the field of computed tomography. Computed tomography involves the use of computer processed x-rays for imaging of the scanned subject. It encompasses a wide range of topics including molecular imaging, development of articulation simulation system with the help of vocal tract model, etc. The aim of this book is to provide distinct information regarding the field of computed tomography to the readers. It will appeal to a great range of readers including researchers, scientists and even students who wish learn more about the technique of computed tomography.

Various studies have approached the subject by analyzing it with a single perspective, but the present book provides diverse methodologies and techniques to address this field. This book contains theories and applications needed for understanding the subject from different perspectives. The aim is to keep the readers informed about the progresses in the field; therefore, the contributions were carefully examined to compile novel researches by specialists from across the globe.

Indeed, the job of the editor is the most crucial and challenging in compiling all chapters into a single book. In the end, I would extend my sincere thanks to the chapter authors for their profound work. I am also thankful for the support provided by my family and colleagues during the compilation of this book.

Editor

Computed Tomography in Abdominal Imaging: How to Gain Maximum Diagnostic Information at the Lowest Radiation Dose

Kristie M. Guite, J. Louis Hinshaw and Fred T. Lee Jr.

Additional information is available at the end of the chapter

1. Introduction

Computed Tomography (CT) was first introduced as a medical device in the 1970's, and has since become a ubiquitous imaging tool. Recent technical advances including faster scan times, improved spatial resolution, and advanced multi-planar reconstruction techniques have led to the application of CT for the evaluation of numerous anatomic abnormalities and disease processes. Approximately 3 million CT scans were performed annually in the United States in 1980, but by 2008 that number had grown to 67 million and it continues to rise. [1] Over two-thirds of all medical radiation is attributable to CT, with 75% of CT scans being performed in the hospital setting. Approximately 40% of CT scans are of the head/neck/spine, 10% of the chest, 47% of the abdomen/pelvis, and the remainder of the extremities or as a procedural tool. [2, 3, 4]

Increasing awareness of medical radiation has paralleled the increase in CT usage with permeation into the popular and scientific press. This has resulted in an emphasis by several organizations on reducing overall medical radiation exposure without compromising diagnostic accuracy and usefulness. Despite this increased awareness and attention, the significance of the increased radiation exposure to the population caused by CT remains unclear. High levels of ionizing radiation exposure are known to increase cancer risk [5, 6, 7] but the data for lower doses of radiation, like those seen during medical imaging (including CT), is less clear and remains controversial. [8, 9, 10] Therefore, in the absence of clarity on this topic, the American College of Radiology (ACR), Health Physics Society (HPS) and other interested organizations have adopted the principles of *As Low As Reasonably Achievable (ALARA)*, *Image Gently* in pediatrics and *Image Wisely* in adults. The common theme of all of these guidelines is to advise physicians to limit radiation exposure to only what is medically necessary. [11, 12]

Several strategies to reduce CT-associated radiation have been attempted. One strategy is to vet CT as the appropriate diagnostic test with preferential use of other imaging modalities such as ultrasound and MRI when able, particularly in pediatrics, and to limit the CT examination to the anatomic area in question. A second strategy involves optimizing scanning parameters (such as kVp, pitch and mA) in order to reduce exposure in all patient populations. [13, 14, 15] If CT is felt to be necessary, applying optimized technical parameters and limiting the scan area can substantially reduce radiation exposure and result in dose reductions as high as 65%. [12, 15] These important techniques are described in other chapters of this book and are not our focus. Rather, we will concentrate on an important, but potentially overlooked source of unnecessary medical radiation, namely, multiphase examinations. We will discuss how multiphasic examination should be used in abdominal imaging with an emphasis on utilizing the minimum number of phases that will suffice for the clinical indication. [16]

1.1. Potential CT phases

The different phases that are possible with state-of-the-art CT scanners are myriad and include scanning before and after contrast administration, delayed imaging, venous and arterial phases, and several others (table 1). Specific patterns of contrast enhancement or evolution of findings over time can dramatically aid in diagnosis in abdominal pathology, thus justifying these additional phases in some patients. However, additional phases should only be necessary in very specific clinical indications, and should be used judiciously as each phase will result in additional radiation. If these additional phases are performed for a specific examination with the same technical parameters as the original phase, which is often the case, the radiation dose is multiplied by the number of phases making it important that the phases performed are clinically indicated and relevant.

Phase		Typical indication	Timing after contrast injection
Non-contrast		Identify calcifications	N/A
Contrast Enhanced			
Angiography		Evaluate vascular anatomy	15-35 sec
Arterial	Early	Arterial structures	15-35 sec
phase	Late	Hypervascular tumors	15-35 sec
Portal venous phase		Majority of routine imaging is performed with this phase. Provides excellent solid organ visualization	60-90 sec
Venous Imaging		Evaluate for venous thrombosis	180 sec
Delayed		Cholangiocarcinoma	10-15 minutes
		Adrenal adenoma	10-15 minutes
		Extravasation (i.e. active bleeding)	7-10 minutes
Renal	Corticomedullary phase	Identification of renal cortical abnormalities	70 sec
	Nephrogenic phase	Characterization and improved visualization of renal masses	100-200 sec
	Excretory phase	Evaluation of the renal collecting system	10 min

Table 1. Common indications for multiphase CT

1.2. Use of multiphasic CT

Multiphase CT examinations are extremely useful in a certain subset of patients. The tempta-tion in a busy practice is to perform CT with a "one size fits all" approach such that physicians will not miss the opportunity to completely characterize even the most unexpected findings. This approach usually means utilizing multiphase scans in all patients to cover multiple potential scenarios. Since most patients do not benefit from additional phases, this practice results in unnecessary radiation in the majority of patients. The dose-multiplication effect of these unnecessary phases can be dramatically reduced or eliminated with individual tailoring of CT exams to the specific clinical scenario. [16]

In an attempt to address this issue, the American College of Radiology (ACR) has developed evidence and expert opinion-based appropriateness criteria matching scanning protocols for various clinical conditions. [17] Unfortunately, the criteria often do not address the most appropriate phase for use in a specific clinical scenario, but rather allude to a "CT Abdomen and Pelvis with IV contrast". Therefore, identification of the most appropriate phases requires a literature review to identify scenarios when additional phases can be expected to add additional useful information. Our approach is to perform single phase imaging (generally the portal venous phase) unless there is specific literature or recommendations to support additional phases. Thus, for the indications addressed by the ACR appropriateness criteria, a portal venous phase is the most likely recommendation. For each indication in the appropri-ateness criteria, the varying imaging modalities are ranked, but they generally do not discuss the use of different phases in CT. They define 1 as being the least appropriate study for the given indication and 9 as being the most appropriate. Similarly, the Royal College of Radiology has also developed guidelines for the same purpose and these guidelines have many similar-ities to, but are not identical to the ACR guidelines [18]. For the purposes of this discussion, we will attempt to describe utilization patterns for CT phases that are supported by the medical literature and while these recommendations are partially based upon the ACR guidelines, we also recommend that physicians become familiar with medical literature supporting the use of multiphasic CT.

1.3. Indications for CT by phase

The majority of CT imaging in the head, chest and extremities are performed with single-phase imaging and won't be specifically addressed. However, abdominal imaging is associated with many potential uses for multiple-phase imaging and will be discussed in detail. The majority of abdominal and pelvic CT's can be performed using a single-phase, but the evaluation of some tumor types (hepatic/pancreatic/renal), the urinary collecting system, and trauma patients among others, may be best performed with multiple phases which is described in more detail below.

In discussing the numerous phases and indications for CT, it should be noted that best patient care requires individualized CT protocols based upon each patient's specific symptoms, pathology, and underlying co-morbidities. Although labor intensive, this provides the highest likelihood of an accurate diagnosis with the lowest necessary radiation dose. The following discussion will provide a basic outline of current best practice, but not all clinical scenarios can be accounted for. Note that the ACR appropriateness criteria can be found on the ACR website (http://www.acr.org/ac).

2. Unenhanced CT

Non-contrast CT scans Figure 1a (left) and 1b (right) are of limited use for the differentiation of soft tissue structures. However, materials like blood, calcium (renal stones, vascular atheroscle-rosis), bone, and pulmonary parenchyma are highly visible and can usually be adequately assessed with non-contrast CT. For example, in the abdomen and pelvis, there are several indications for non-contrast imaging. These include: evaluation of renal calculi; assessment for gross intra-abdominal hemorrhage; and post-endostent volume measurements. In addition, non-contrast images are often obtained in conjunction with contrast enhanced images in evaluating potential renal transplant donors and in the evaluation of the pancreas (in combina-tion with contrast phases). Of note, dual-energy CT and the development of virtual "non-contrast" images may ultimately obviate the combination scans. Additionally, CT angiography examinations performed for pathologies like aneurysms and dissection are frequently per-formed in conjunction with non-contrast imaging. The non-contrast images facilitate the differentiation of active extravasation or acute bleeding from vascular calcifications.

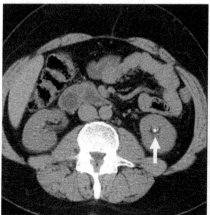 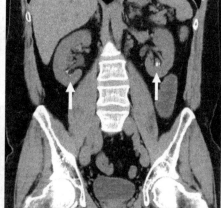

Figure 1. Non-contrast CT demonstrating multiple bilateral renal calculi (arrows), which can be obscured on contrast-enhanced images, particularly delayed images when there is excreted contrast in the renal collecting system; axial left, coronal reformat on right.

3. Contrast-enhanced CT

Contrast enhanced CT examinations can be acquired at a variety of specific time points after intravenous contrast injection (timing is dependent on the phase of contrast enhancement needed and organ system being evaluated). The timing should be chosen specifically to optimize contrast distribution within the solid organ parenchyma in question.

3.1. Portal venous phase

The most common technique is to perform portal venous phase imaging in the abdomen and pelvis (approximately 60-90 seconds after contrast administration, figure 2). This results in near optimal contrast opacification of the majority of the solid abdominal organs and it is used for a wide variety of indications: nonspecific abdominal pain; hernia; infection; masses (with a few exceptions such as hypervascular, renal, and some hepatic tumors); and in most follow-up examinations. As a general rule, this single phase is adequate unless there is a specific clinical indication that has been shown to benefit from other phases.

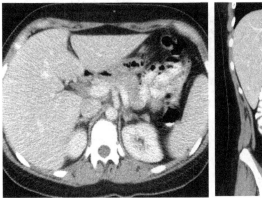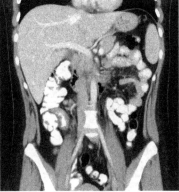

Figure 2. Contrast enhanced CT demonstrating parenchymal enhancement of the intra-abdominal organs in the portal venous phase (axial left, coronal reformat right).

3.2. Early arterial phase (CT Angiography (CTA))

CT angiography (CTA) is highly effective for evaluation of the arterial system, and has largely replaced conventional angiography due to the lower risk profile and ability to survey the entire abdomen. Images are acquired after a rapid bolus of intravenous contrast material (3-7 cc/s) during the arterial phase (15-35 seconds after injection) when the concentration of contrast material in the arterial system is high (figures 3). Images are usually acquired using narrow collimation (<1 mm) and can be retrospectively reconstructed using dedicated 3-dimensional workstations and software. CTA is commonly used in the head and chest in the evaluation of pulmonary emboli, aneurysms, vascular malformations, dissection, bleeding and ischemia. Indications for early arterial phase imaging include: evaluation of aneurysms or dissections (cerebral, aortic, etc.), hepatic, splanchnic or renal arterial anatomy, and arterial imaging in liver or kidney transplantation. Single phase arterial imaging is often used in the evaluation of trauma patients either a complete chest/abdomen/pelvis examination with arterial phase imaging of the chest and portal venous phase imaging of the abdomen/pelvis or just a portal venous phase of abdomen and pelvis depending on the mechanism and severity of the trauma. CTA is also commonly performed in the abdomen and pelvis for evaluating vascular malformations and in the evaluation of bleeding. Mesenteric ischemia can also be evaluated using CT angiography. CTA of the abdomen and pelvis is often performed in combination with a CTA for evaluating the extremity vasculature.

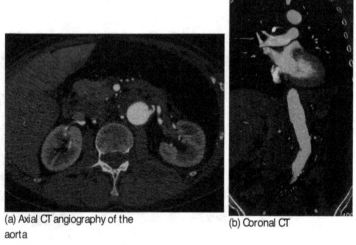

(a) Axial CT angiography of the aorta

(b) Coronal CT

Figure 3. Axial (left) and coronal (right) CT angiography images of the abdominal aorta evaluating for aortic aneurysm.

3.3. Late arterial phase

The late arterial phase is timed to correspond to the peak concentration of contrast material in highly vascular tumors and is performed approximately 20-35 seconds after the injection of intravenous contrast. Early arterial phase imaging is predominantly utilized for angiography and will be discussed separately. Late arterial phase imaging is almost always performed in conjunction with other phases (e.g. portal venous phase) to allow more complete characterization of any identified abnormalities (figure 4). The primary indication for a late arterial phase is for the evaluation of hypervascular tumors of the liver such as hepatocellular carcinoma or hypervascular metastases (figure 4). Typical hypervascular tumors for which this would be used include: hepatocellular carcinoma; renal cell carcinoma; melanoma; carcinoid/neuroendocrine tumors; some sarcomas; choriocarcinoma; and thyroid carcinoma. Although a "hypervascular", biphasic evaluation would generally be used for these patients, note that a single phase is often adequate for follow up imaging.

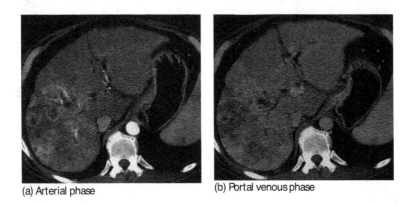

(a) Arterial phase   (b) Portal venous phase

Figure 4. Selected images from a biphasic CT demonstrating early arterial enhancement of a posterior right hepatic lobe mass with mild wash out on delayed phase images in the setting of cirrhosis characteristic of hepatocellular carcinoma.

3.4. Systemic venous phase imaging

CT imaging specific for the venous structures is performed uncommonly. Most venous structures are partially opacified on the routine contrast enhancing images and suffice for most examinations. However, occasionally evaluation of the inferior vena cava is desired, such as prior to IVC filter placement/removal or evaluation of IVC thrombosis.

3.5. Delayed phase

Delayed phase imaging (figure 5) encompasses scanning at a variety of different times following contrast administration, and depends on the pathology in question. Typical delayed imaging times range from a few minutes to up to 15 minutes or longer. The most common indications for delayed phase imaging are evaluation of the kidneys, collecting system (ureters and bladder) and specific kidney, liver, and adrenal tumors. [19, 20] Evaluation of the kidneys, ureters and bladder are discussed separately in the renal imaging section. Cholangiocarcinoma occurring within the extrahepatic biliary tree or intrahepatic cholangiocarcinomas are a common reason for delayed imaging. Cholangiocarcinomas are fibrotic tumors which enhance slowly, and are usually imaged following a 10-15 minute delay. Similarly, adrenal masses can be evaluated with multiphase imaging including an unenhanced CT, portal venous phase and a 10 minute delay CT which allows for evaluation and calculation of the enhancement and washout characteristics aiding in distinguishing benign adrenal adenomas from other adrenal masses.

Outside of the evaluation of masses, delayed phase images can be used in the evaluation of active vascular extravasation in trauma patients, vascular malformations, and aneurysm disruption.

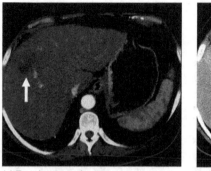 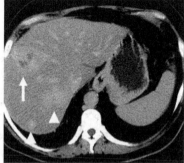

(a) Portal venous phase   (b) Portal venous phase

Figure 5. Selected images form CT performed using a Cholangiocarcinoma specific protocol. 5a is a portal venous phase image demonstrating a single low attenuation mass which does not appear to enhance. 5b is a 15 minute delayed image which demonstrates delayed enhancement of the liver mass (arrow) characteristic of Cholangiocarcinoma. Several other enhancing masses (arrowheads) are also seen which were not evident on the portal venous phase images.

4. Organ specific considerations

4.1. Hepatic masses

When evaluating hepatic masses, it can be advantageous to have both late arterial and portal venous phase images (biphasic imaging, figure 4) since some tumors enhance briskly during the arterial phase (hepatocellular carcinoma, hepatic adenoma, follicular nodular hyperplasia (FNH), and hypervascular metastasis), but may be occult or difficult to characterize on portal venous phase imaging alone (figure 6). However, it should be stressed that the addition of late arterial phase images is only indicated if one of these tumors is suspected, or if there is a need for further characterization of a hepatic mass, since the large majority of patients will not benefit from the addition of this phase. In addition, if there is a need to definitively characterize a hepatic mass, MRI is generally more sensitive and specific, with no associated radiation dose.

4.2. Renal masses

Detection and characterization of renal parenchymal masses is a frequent indication for CT. An initial noncontrast CT is important for detecting calcium or fat in a lesion, and to provide baseline attenuation of any renal masses. Following noncontrast scanning, intravenous contrast is injected and a corticomedullary phase is obtained at approximately 70 seconds (figure 7a, 7b). The corticomedullary phase is characterized by enhancement of the renal cortex as well as the renal vasculature. This phase is valuable in the evaluation of benign renal variants, lymphadenopathy and vasculature, however certain medullary renal masses may not be visible during this phase due to minimal enhancement of the medulla and collecting

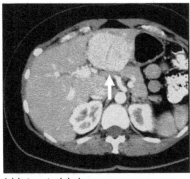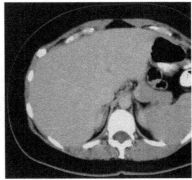

(a) Late arterial phase   (b) Portal venous phase

Figure 6. Selected images from a biphasic CT of Focal Nodular Hyperplasia in the left hepatic lobe (arrow). These masses have characteristic early arterial enhancement (6a) with contrast wash out on the portal venous phase images (6b) from the mass making these lesions difficult to identify on portal venous phase images alone.

system. The parenchymal phase is obtained approximately 100-200 seconds after the injection of contrast material (figure 7c). Parenchymal phase imaging demonstrates continued enhancement of the cortex, enhancement of the medulla, and various levels of contrast material in the collecting system. The parenchymal phase is highly important for the detection and characterization of renal masses, parenchymal abnormalities, and the renal collecting system. [21] This method of imaging does not evaluate for abnormalities of the collecting system.

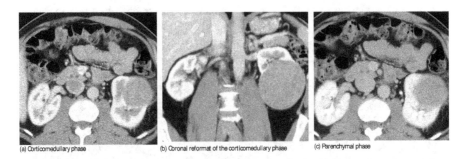

(a) Corticomedullary phase   (b) Coronal reformat of the corticomedullary phase   (c) Parenchymal phase

Figure 7. Selected images from a renal mass specific protocol CT. Corticomedullary phase (axial 7a) demonstrates peripheral enhancement of the renal cortex with minimal opacification of the renal medulla. There is a large renal cell carcinoma in the right kidney which can be differentiated from the normal renal parenchyma by the heterogeneous and differential enhancement. The renal artery and vein are opacified in this phase as well. The collecting system is not opacified (coronal reformat 7b). In the parenchymal phase, the renal cortex and the medulla are enhancing. The renal cell carcinoma in the left kidney is not as well defined when compared to the corticomedullary phase images, but is actually slightly more conspicuous. There is some contrast noted within the collecting system during this phase (7c).

Common renal masses can occasionally be differentiated from each other using this imaging technique. Renal cell carcinomas and oncocytomas typically demonstrate intense heterogeneous enhancement on the parenchymal phase images and cannot be reliably differentiated from each other but can be distinguished from other renal masses. Angiomyolipomas (AML's) also demonstrate intense contrast enhancement but characteristically contain macroscopic fat which can be detected on the noncontrast images, and can help to differentiate AML's from renal cell carcinomas and oncocytomas. Renal lymphoma on the other hand, will often have decreased enhancement when compared to the renal parenchyma on the parenchymal phase images.

4.3. CT urography

CT urography (CTU) is commonly used in the evaluation of hematuria, and specifically tailored to image the renal collecting system, ureters and bladder in addition to the renal parenchyma. Initial imaging includes a noncontrast phase to detect renal calculi as a source of hematuria. Note that dual energy CT may eventually allow the noncontrast phase to be eliminated. Contrast enhancement techniques for CTU vary from institution to institution. A common technique used at our institution and others is a double bolus, single phase imaging algorithm. This technique is a hybrid contrast injection strategy that results in opacification of the renal parenchyma (parenchymal phase, figure 8a) and the collecting system, ureters, and bladder (excretory phase, figure 8b and 8c). At our institution, a small contrast bolus is administered initially, followed 10 minutes later with a larger bolus that is imaged in the corticomedullary phase. This ensures that contrast is being excreted by the kidneys and thus the collecting system is opacified (excretory phase) from the initial injection, and that the renal parenchyma is enhancing as well from the second injection (parenchymal phase). At the conclusion of the urography protocol, we also perform a scout image in the supine and prone position to allow a global evaluation of the collecting system. Excretory phase imaging allows for not only evaluation of the ureteral lumen, but also periureteral abnormalities including external masses and lymphadenopathy. [22]

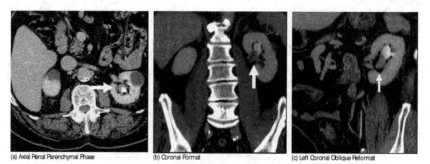

(a) Axial Renal Parenchymal Phase   (b) Coronal Format   (c) Left Coronal Oblique Reformat

Figure 8. Selected images from a CT Urography protocol CT. 8a is an axial CT image from the renal parenchymal phase. There is a mildly enhancing soft tissue mass in the left renal pelvis (arrow) consistent with a transitional cell carcinoma. Figure 8b (coronal reformats) and 8c (left oblique coronal reformats) demonstrate the double bolus technique of CT Urography. These images confirm soft tissue mass (arrows) in the renal pelvis with contrast excretion into the collecting system (arrowheads).

4.4. Pancreatic masses

Pancreatic masses are often evaluated using both an early arterial (to evaluate for vascular involvement and thus resectability, figure 9a) and a later "pancreatic" phase (which optimizes pancreatic parenchymal enhancement and thus is best at differentiating pancreatic tumors from pancreatic parenchyma, figure 9b). Pancreatic adenocarcinoma typically is hypoenhancing when compared to the surrounding parenchyma. Most other common pancreatic tumors are hypervascular with avid enhancement (such as pancreatic neuroendocrine tumors) and appear brighter than the surrounding pancreatic parenchyma after the injection of intravenous contrast material.

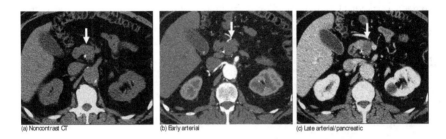

(a) Noncontrast CT (b) Early arterial (c) Late arterial/pancreatic

Figure 9. Selected images from a pancreatic protocol. 9a is a noncontrast CT image demonstrating subtle fullness in the region of the pancreatic neck (arrow). 9b is a CT image performed during the early arterial phase during which there is opacification of the arterial structure with subtle fullness in the pancreatic neck (arrow). The pancreas is not enhancing during this phase. 9c was performed in a late arterial/pancreatic phase demonstrating normal enhancement of the pancreas (arrowhead) with a hypoenhancing mass (arrow) in the pancreatic neck. The pancreatic mass is more visible during this phase.

4.5. Incidental findings

CT imaging should be performed to evaluate the specific clinical question, however incidental findings are noted in approximately 5-16 % of patients scanned for an unrelated reasons. [23, 24] It is not acceptable practice to anticipate the possibility of incidental lesions given their low incidence and prospectively add additional phases to routine protocols. Unfortunately, several recent surveys demonstrated that this practice is more common than might be anticipated, and contributes to unnecessary medical radiation exposure to a large population of patients. [16] Even more egregious is the fact that many of these findings could potentially be more accurately evaluated with other non-radiation imaging modalities such as MRI or ultrasound.

Although the management of incidental findings is not the focus of this chapter, some of these findings will require complete characterization with further CT phases such as arterial phase (certain liver tumors) or delayed images (adrenal lesions). Management of incidental findings has been controversial since they are relatively common, especially in the elderly, and more CT scanning may be required for further characterization of what is frequently a benign finding. In an effort to provide guidance on which incidental findings should be appropriately further evaluated and what the appropriate imaging modality should be, the ACR published a white paper on management of incidental findings detected at CT of the abdomen in 2010. [25]

5. Conclusion

Multiphase CT examinations are very important for the detection and characterization of certain clinical conditions, but should not be generalized for every patient undergoing CT of the abdomen and pelvis. A recent survey demonstrated that many physicians are routinely performing multiphase CT for the majority of patients in an attempt to prospectively characterize potential lesions detected during the scan. However, unindicated multiphase CT examinations are an important source of medical radiation that does not contribute to the care of patients. Adherence to published standards such as the ACR Appropriateness Criteria can both decrease medical radiation and optimize imaging for the specific clinical indication.

Abbreviations

1. CT (computed tomography)

2. kVp (Kilovoltage)

3. ma (Milliamperes)

4. CTA (Computed Tomography Angiography)

5. CTU (Computed Tomography Urography)

6. MRI (Magnetic Resonance Imaging)

7. ACR (American College of Radiology)

Author details

Kristie M. Guite, J. Louis Hinshaw* and Fred T. Lee Jr.

*Address all correspondence to: jhinshaw@uwhealth.org

Department of Radiology, University of Wisconsin, Madison, WI, USA

References

[1] Gazelle, Scott G, Halpern, et al.Utilization of Diagnostic Medical Imaging: Comparison of Radiologist Referral versus Same-Specialty Referral.*Radiology*, 2007;245(2): 517-522.

[2] Brenner, DJ, Hall EJ.Computed Tomography – An Increasing Source of Radiation Exposure.*NEJM*, 2007;357:2277-2284.

[3] Mettler FA Jr, Wiest PW, Locken JA, Kelsey CA.CT Scanning : Pattern of Use and Dose.*Journal of Radiological Protection*, 2000;204:353 -359.

[4] Brix G, Nissen-Meyer S, Lechel U, et al.Radiation exposures of Cancer Patients from Medical X-rays: How Relevant are they for Individual Patients and Population Exposure?*European Journal of Radiology*, 2009;72(2):342-347.

[5] Pierce DA, Preston, DL.Radiation-Related Cancer Risks at Low Doses Among Atomic Bomb Survivors.*Radiat Res*, 2000;154:178-186.

[6] Pierce DA, Shimizu Y, Preston DL, Vaeth M., Mabuchi K.Studies of the Mortality of Atomic Bomb Survivors.Report 12, Part I.Cancer- 1950-1990.*Radiation Res*, 1996;146:1-27.

[7] Muirhead CR.Studies on the Hiroshima and Nagasaki Survivors, and Their Use in Estimating Radiation Risks.*Radiation Protection Dosimetry*, 2003;104:331-335.

[8] Mezerich R.Are CT Scans Carcinogenic?*American College of Radiology*, 2008:691-693.

[9] Cardis E, Vrijheid M, Blettner M, et al.Risk of Cancer After Low Doses of Ionizing Radiation: Retrospective Cohort Study in 15 Countries.*BMJ*, 2005; 331-377.

[10] Little MP, Wakeford R, Tawn JE, Bouffler SD, Berrington de Gonzalez A.Risks Associated with Low Doses and Low Dose rates of Ionizing radiation: Why Linearity May be (Almost) the Best We Can Do.*Radiology*, 2009;251(1):6-12.

[11] Committee on the Biological Effects of Ionizing Radiation.Health Effects of Exposure to Low Levels of Ionizing Radiation.Washington, DC: National academy Press, 1990.

[12] ICRP.1990 Recommendations of the International Commission on Radiological Protection.ICRP Publication no 60.Oxford, UK:Pergamon, 1991.

[13] Tack D, De Maertelaer V, Gevenois PA.Dose Reduction in Multidetector CT Using Attenuation-Based Online Tube Current Modulation. *American Journal of Roentgenology*, 2003;181:331-334.

[14] Paterson A, Frush D, Donnelly LF.Helical CT of the Body : Are Settings Adjusted for Pediatric Patients?*American Journal of Radiology*, 2001;176: 297-301.

[15] Greess H, Nomayr A, Wolf H, Baum U, et al.Dose Reduction in CT Examinations of Children by an attenuation-based on-line modulation of tube current(CARE dose).*European Radiology*, 2002;12:1571-1576.

[16] Guite, KM, Hinshaw, JL, Ranallo, FN, Lindstrom, MJ, Lee, FT.Ionizing Radiation in Abdominal Computed Tomography: UnindicatedMuliphase Scans are an Important Source of Medically Unnecessary Exposure.*JACR* 2011;8:756-761.

[17] ACR Appropriateness Criteria 2008.Available at: http://acr.org/acr.

[18] Royal College of Radiologists. Making the best use of clinical radiology services: re-
      ferral guidelines. 6th ed. London: Royal College of Radiologists; 2007.

[19] Boland GW, Hahn PF, Pena C, Mueller PR. Adrenal masses: characterization with
      delayed contrast-enhanced CT. *Radiology* 1997; 202:693-696.

[20] Lacomis JM, Baron RL, Oliver JH 3rd, Nalesnik MA, Federle MP. Cholangiocarcino-
      ma: delayed CT contrast enhancement patterns. 1997;;203(1):98-104.

[21] Szolar DH, Kammerhuber F, Altzieber S, et al. Multiphasic helical CT of the kidney:
      increased conspicuity for detectionand characterization of small (<3 cm) renal mass-
      es. *Radiology* 1997; 201:211-217

[22] Caoili EM, Inampudi P, Cohan RH, etal.MDCTU of upper tract uroepithelial malig-
      nancy. *Am J Roentgenol* 2003; 180:71.

[23] Pickhardt PJ, Hanson ME, Vanness DJ, et al. Unsuspectedextracolonic findings at
      screening CT colonography: clinical and economic impact. *Radiology* 2008;249:151-9.

[24] Hassan C, Pickhardt PJ, Laghi A, et al. Computed tomographic colonography to
      screen for colorectal cancer, extracolonic cancer, and aortic aneurysm: model simula-
      tion with cost-effectiveness analysis. *Arch Intern* Med 2008;168:696-705.

[25] Berland LL, Silverman SG, Gore RM, Mayo-Smith WW, Megibow AJ, Yee J, Brink JA,
      Baker ME, Federle MP, Foley WD, Francis IR, Herts BR, Israel GM, Krinsky G, Platt
      JF, Shuman WP, Taylor AJ. Managing Incidental Findings on Abdominal CT: White
      Paper of the ACR Incidental Findings Committee.*J Am CollRadiol* 2010;7:754-773.

Chapter 2

Molecular Imaging

Fathinul Fikri Ahmad Saad, Abdul Jalil Nordin,
Hishar Hassan, Cheah Yoke Kqueen and W.F.E Lau

Additional information is available at the end of the chapter

1. Introduction

Molecular imaging techniques depend upon molecular mechanisms operative in vivo. This imaging technique encompasses the visualization, characterization and measurement of biological processes at the molecular and cellular levels in humans and other living systems [1]. The techniques used include Positron Emission Tomography – Computed Tomography (PET-CT), nuclear medicine, Magnetic Resonance Imaging (MRI), Magnetic Resonance Spectroscopy (MRS), optical imaging and ultrasound.

There are escalating evidences in the published data that discussed the advantages of integrated molecular imaging technique as an accurate tool in localizing abnormal metabolic alteration and serve as a potential role as an invasive surrogate biomarker for various disease entities [2,3,4,5]. It also plays an increasingly fundamental role in drug discovery and early development in humans. The evolution of molecular imaging tool in specific PET-CT has impacted the use of molecular imaging technique in many altered cellular mechanism. In particular, PET which was introduced in the 1970 s is capable of quantifying individual changes on the different pathology that underpin the biological reprogramming in abnormal cells [6]. Intensive research activities in various PET applications gradually evolved to its clinical use first in neuropsychiatric disorders and cardiology, then in oncology.

Molecular imaging provides the key to the future of personalized medicine, which involves diagnosing, treating and monitoring patients based on their individual makeup. The amelioration in its technique has braced the one-stop-imaging strategy in various disease entities as a tool for disease localization, prediction and treatment monitoring. For the purpose of the discussion in this chapter, we highlight the integrated molecular imaging technique PET-CT employing flurodeoxyglucose (FDG) as a standard of care utility in various disease pathology.

2. Types of molecular imaging techniques

Molecular imaging, a new discipline in biomedical research has increasingly become a vital tool in disease diagnostic frontier. It offers an excellent visualization, characterization and quantification of biologic process taking place at the cellular and sub-cellular levels. As of now, there are four main categories of molecular imaging modalities; ultrasound, optical imaging, magnetic resonance imaging (MRI), and nuclear imaging techniques (Table 1). Bonekamp [7] in his paper reported that the selection of the imaging modality often is determined based on the temporal and spatial resolution, field of view, sensitivity of the imaging system, depth of the biological process, the molecular or cellular process to image, and the availability of suitable probes and labels than can be delivered to the imaging target. An overview of mechanism behind each of the modalities will be covered in the subsequent section.

Molecular Imaging Modalities	
Single modality	Multimodalities
Ultrasound	PET-CT
MRI	SPECT-CT
PET	PET-MRI
SPECT	
Optical Imaging	

Table 1. Types of Molecular Imaging Modalities

2.1. Ultrasound

Ultrasound imaging has been used for over 20 years. It uses high-frequency sound waves to view soft tissues such as muscles and internal organs inside the body. As the image of the ultrasound is captured in real-time, it enables the physician to see the movement of the body's internal organs as well as blood flowing through the vessels. In an ultrasound exam, a hand-held transducer is placed against the skin. The transducer sends out high frequency sound waves that reflect off the body structures. As sound waves directed through the body bounce back when they encounter different tissues, echoes are measured with the help of a computer and are converted into real-time images of organs and tissues. The image captured is based on the frequency and strength of the sound signal and the time it takes to return from the patient to the transducer [8].

2.2. Optical imaging

In optical imaging, light-producing proteins are designed to attach to specific molecules such as brain chemicals or molecules on the surface of cancer cells [9]. Highly sensitive detectors are employed for detection of low levels of light emitted by specific molecules from inside the body. The two major types of optical imaging are bioluminescent imaging and fluorescence imaging. Bioluminescent imaging uses a natural light-emitting protein to trace the movement of certain cells or to identify the location of specific chemical reactions within the body. In contrast, fluorescence imaging uses proteins that produce light when activated by an external light source such as laser.

2.3. Magnetic resonance imaging

Magnetic resonance imaging or popularly known as MRI is an imaging technique used mainly in medical settings to produce high quality images of inside human body. Theoretically, the mechanism behind MRI is based on the principles of nuclear magnetic resonance (NMR), a spectroscopic technique used by scientist to obtain microscopic chemical and physical information about molecules [10]. MRI scanner has a tube surrounded by a giant circular magnet. During routine examination of MRI, patient is placed on a moveable bed that is inserted into the magnet. The presence of magnet creates a strong magnetic field that aligns the protons of hydrogen atoms, which are then exposed to a beam of radio waves [11]. This spins various protons of the body, and produces a faint signal that is detected by the receiver portion of the MRI scanner. The receiver information is processed by a computer and an image is then produced.

2.4. Nuclear Imaging

Nuclear imaging or also called as radionuclide scanning provides an effective diagnostic tools for the radiologists as it shows not only the structure of an organ but also the function of the organ. Nuclear imaging routine uses small amounts of radioactive material, or tracer for diagnostic purpose. Radioactive tracer used in nuclear imaging is normally a specifically targeted probe. It could be antibodies, ligands or substrates to specifically interact with protein targets in particular cells or sub cellular compartments. These interactions are based on either receptor-radioligand binding or enzyme mediated trapping of a radio labeled substrate [12]. Radioactive tracers used in nuclear imaging are in most cases is administered into a vein and some are given orally. After an administration of radioactive tracers, patient is required to rest for a certain period to allow distribution of radioactive tracer in the body. In the end, for imaging purpose, a specialized gamma camera is used to detect the radiation throughout the body. Most commonly used techniques in nuclear imaging are positron emission tomography (PET) and single photon emission computed tomography (SPECT).

2.4.1. Positron Emission Tomography (PET)

Positron emission tomography or known as 'PET' is a rapidly developing nuclear imaging technique, with a clinical role that now exceeds almost 15 years [13]. It is a quantitative tomographic imaging technique which produces cross-sectional images that are composites of volume elements [14]. The signal intensity for PET images in each voxel is dependent upon the activity of radionuclide tagged with radioactive tracer which intravenously adminis-tered at the earlier stage before the scanning takes place. A scanner which usually called PET scanner employs a gamma photon coincidence detection system designed for oppositely directed annihilation photons emitted indirectly by the positron decay of PET radionuclides. This logic allows acquisition of images that are quantitative three dimensional (3-D) maps of radiolabeled tracers in tissue. The most commonly used PET radioactive tracer is the glucose derivative, 2-[^{18}F]fluoro-2-deoxy-D-glucose or commercially known as [^{18}F]FDG, with numerous other tracers under development capable of highlighting a broad range of organ and tissue metabolic functions. In a large meta-analysis, PET was shown to change management in 30% of patients [15].

2.4.2. Single Photon Emission Computed Tomography (SPECT)

Similar to PET, single photon emission computed tomography (SPECT) also uses a radioactive tracer that is administered to the patient and a scanner to record data that a computer constructs into two or three dimensional images. However, in another note, SPECT technique employs a gamma camera that rotates around the patient to detect a radioactive tracer in the body. In contrast to PET which employs shorter half-lived tracers as opposed to the SPECT tracers [16]. If a tumor is present, the antibodies will stick to it and thus allow for detection of tumorous cells. For better understanding on strength and weakness of each imaging modalities, Table 2 below provides a summary of the imaging techniques with its respective strength and weakness.

Imaging modality	Electro magnetic radiation spectrum	Advantages	Disadvantages
Ultrasound	High-frequency sound	Real time and low cost	Limited spatial resolution, mostly morphologic although targeted micro bubbles under development
Optical bioluminescence imaging	Visible light	Highest sensitivity, quick, easy, low cost and relatively high throughput	Low spatial resolution, current 2-D imaging only, relatively surface weighted, limited translational research
Optical fluorescence imaging	Visible light or near-infrared	High sensitivity, detects fluorochrome in live and dead cells	Relatively low spatial resolution, relatively surface weighted
Magnetic resonance imaging (MRI)	Radio waves	Highest spatial resolution, combines morphologic and functional imaging	Relatively low sensitivity, long scan and post processing time, mass quantity of probe may be needed
Positron Emission Tomography (PET)	High energy gamma rays	High sensitivity, shorter time scan, enable quantitative analysis	PET cyclotron or generator needed, relatively low spatial resolution
Single photon emission computed tomography (SPECT)	Lower energy gamma rays	Many molecular probes available, can image multiple probes simultaneously, may be adapted to clinical imaging system	Relatively low spatial resolution, high radiation to subjects due to longer tracer half-life's, non-quantitative tool, Longer scanning time

Table 2. Key strength and weakness of the main available imaging modalities used in molecular imaging [12, 16]

3. Integrated molecular imaging techniques (FDG PET-CT)

The astonishing achievement of the molecular imaging technique rely on its ability to signal altered metabolism in a targeted pathological cells whereby two imaging modalities are integrated in a single setting (multimodality imaging technique/integrated imaging) i.e. PET-CT, SPECT-CT, PET-MRI. It includes two- or three-dimensional imaging as well as quantification over time (Figure 1). Largely independent of structural disturbances, integrated molecular imaging techniques increasingly offer high spatial resolution, but more particularly, high contrast. Minute quantities of radioactive materials, chosen because of their ability to participate in biological processes of interest, can provide highly sensitive indications of body function in health and disease. Therefore, disordered metabolism or physiology can be detected with high sensitivity and the anatomical distribution of abnormality can be determined with greater precision than the conventional technique (Table 3). The conventional imaging techniques i.e. computed tomography (CT) or standalone nuclear medicine technique – single positron emission tomography (SPECT) are relatively unpopular in a current scenario given their limitations to only evaluating the structural changes or functional changes disjointedly.

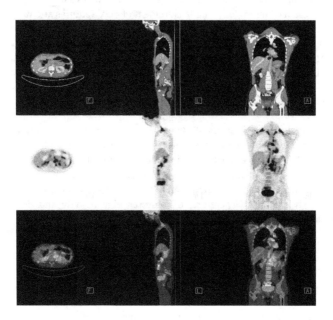

Figure 1. PET-CT image display on the Syngo console panel showing series of CT, PET and fused images.

Published data	Sensitivity versus Specificity (%)	
	PET-CT	CT
Niikura N et al Metastatic breast cancer[2]	97.4 versus 91.2	85.9 versus 67.3
Kim SK et al (solitary pulmonary lesion)[3]	97.0 versus 85	93.0 versus 31.0
Pim A. et al (malignant lymphoma)[4]	100.0versus 95.0	91.0 versus 96.0
Ozkan E et al (colorectal cancer recurrence) [5]	98.0 versus 85.0	73.0 versus 86.0

Table 3. Data shows the accuracy of the PET-Ct and the CT in the evaluation of various tumors

3.1. FDG PET-CT and Standard Uptake Value (SUV)

The imaging of the alteration of the glucose metabolism, as reflected by cellular uptake and trapping of the glucose analog 18F-FDG can suffice a response assessment that is both accurate and contemporaneously than that provided by standard morphologic imaging. Quantitative evaluation of FDG PET images provides quantitative data in the form of the standardized uptake value (SUV). This is an uptake measurement that provides a mean of comparison of FDG uptake between different lesions. Measurement of SUV requires attenuation correction to avoid the variability in FDG uptake due to the differences in tumor habitus within the body. This value normalizes the tumor FDG uptake with the FDG injected activity and the body weight [17]. The cut-off value of 2.5 in differentiating malignant to benign is at large limited due to varied tumor histological characteristic in malignant tumor [18]

3.2. FDG PET-CT and radiation issues

Being a glucose analogue, 2-[^{18}F]fluoro-2-deoxy-D-glucose or commonly known as ^{18}F-FDG, is the most commonly used positron emitting radiopharmaceutical in PET examination. The preparation of ^{18}F-FDG involves the production of radioisotope fluorine-18 to tag with glucose derivative. Fluorine-18, a positron emitters, emits gamma energy of 511 keV and due to positron annihilation, it emits total energy of 1022 keV. This is almost 10 times higher than conventional X-ray radiation. Therefore, it possesses high activity and dose exposure to radiation workers and patients.

However, the radiation exposure could be outweighed due to its benefit to the patient. This is in compliance with the International Commission on Radiological Protection (ICRP) which recommended three elements in the system of dose limitation [19]. The three elements are; justification, optimization and dose limitation. Justification means that any propose examina-tion that may cause exposure to the patients should yield a sufficient benefit to the patients to justify the risk incurred by the radiation exposure. This element is based on the assumption that any radiation exposure, either it is in small dose, carries with it a certain level of risk that is proportional to the level of exposure. The second element is optimization, which is also known as the practice of ALARA (as low as reasonably achievable). This by all means, the radiation exposures resulting from the examination or preparation of radiopharmaceuticals must be reduced to the lowest level possible, considering the cost of such a reduction in dose. The third element in ICRP recommendation is dose limitation. The dose limits are normally imposed by the local regulatory agencies.

To accommodate a dose exposure at minimum, certain laboratory technique can be improved when dealing with radioactive materials. The use of teleplier, long tong or robotic arms can maximize the distance between the radioactive material and personnel. This directly reduces the dose expose to the radiation worker [20]. In the administrative and procedure control aspect, the introduction of automated dose dispensing will replace the manual dose dispensing activity performs by the radiation worker to eliminate receiving of unnecessary exposure. The rotation between personnel involves in preparation of radiopharmaceutical and examination also provides an alternative way to reduce high dose expose. Nevertheless, PET utilizes ^{18}F-FDG as a radiotracer carries a low absorbed dose to patient estimated at approximately 7 mSv. The radiation (x rays) from our diagnostic CT protocol ranges from 8mSv to 16 mSv. The new technology 64 multislice CT technique is equipped with the dual focal spot that ensures more image yields without increased in the total radiation dose. The modulated tube current adaptation of higher multislice CT scanner (64 and above) technique as offered by many vendors is capable of reducing patient dose up to 20% as compared to the lower 16 multislice of the same kind. [21,22]. In a nutshell, even though the use of molecular imaging modalities possesses risk onto the patients and radiation workers, but the purpose of examination outweigh the implication of the dose receive and it offers benefit for diagnosis and treatment purpose.

4. Molecular imaging in clinical application

4.1. Utility of integrated molecular imaging (PET-CT) in oncology

Oncology is now the most important application of molecular imaging techniques i.e. PET [23]. In oncology, PET can be used for signaling biological process that underpins pathological reprogramming that promotes carcinogenesis. Among the important signaling processes involved are the altered glucose metabolism, amino acid metabolism, cell membranes metabolism and cell proliferation (Figure 2). Leveraging the rapidly increasing pace of technological and scientific innovation in molecular biology, there has been a surge in the understanding of the key drivers of malignant transformation. An important key driver in malignant transformation is the altered glucose metabolism whereby a glucose analog or Flurodeoxyglucose (FDG) has been utilized as a popular ligand used in labeling the tumor targets.

In vivo, intense FDG uptake and metabolism of glucose, a frequent characteristic of most cancer cells, is associated with an alteration in the intrinsic energy metabolism causing a shift from oxidative phosphorylation to aerobic glycolysis, a change referred to as the Warburg effect [24]. Otto Warburg, working in Germany in the 1920s, discovered that cancer cells have a characteristically increased glycolysis even under aerobic conditions. Because glycolysis is considerably less efficient than oxidative phosphorylation at producing adenosine triphosphate (ATP), the tumor cell requires acceleration in the rate of glucose uptake and use. Given the known

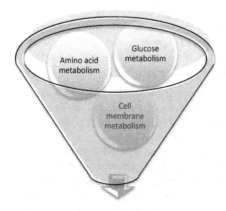

Figure 2. Biomarker signalling in a cell model 18F-FDG : Glucose metabolism, 18F-FET(fluoroethyltyrosine): amino acid metabolism, 18F-FCH(18F-fluorocholine): cell membrane metabolism

natural behaviours of tumors, [18F] FDG accumulation in tumors is used as index of increased glucose metabolism and as a marker of tumor viability for which, the degree of [18F] FDG uptake usually reflects tumor aggressiveness. The kinetics of the FDG tracers is similar to glucose. It passes through the brain-blood barrier and is phosphorylated intracellularly in a process analogous to the glucose. The phosphorylized FDG compound does not enter in the Krebs cycle, thence it is effectively trapped. FDG as a molecular marker in signifying the molecular pathways of each cancer types in different types of cancer of the study. Malignant cells have increased facilitated glucose transport and up regulation of hexokinase activity, and hence tumors can be identified by regions of increased glucose utilization [25]. The PET tracer FDG, a glucose analog, is used to image glucose metabolism in patients. Focal areas of abnormally increased FDG uptake are considered suspicious for malignant disease, particularly as metabolic changes often precede the morphological changes associated with disease. Heterogeneity of malignant cell clones in different sites within a single tumor and between different tumor sites in the body is a manifestation of the genomic instability that characterizes cancer cells [26]. Among the indication for PET-CT in oncology is shown in table 4.

Tumour localisation
Pretreatment tumour staging
Prognostic stratification
Treatment monitoring
Tumour surveillance and restaging
Radiation treatment planning
Development of new anticancer drugs

Table 4. Common indications of PET-CT study

4.2. FDG PET-CT in tumor localisation

By integrating two imaging modalities encompassing the structural and functional imaging techniques, a substantial change in the treatment planning can be achieved while reducing the cost burden and averting futile treatment to patients. Contrasted CT technique used for the evaluation of equivocal PET results promises higher achievable diagnostic results in the assessment of neuroendocrine tumor with prevalence brown fat accumulation. [27]. Furthermore, the details of the surrounding vitals structures are shown clearly on the co registered contrasted CT image for appropriate correlation with the high metabolic focus on PET [28]. The impact of PET in detecting diffuse involvement of other organ system as part of the metastatic spread or delineation of subcentimetre focus of FDG-avidity i.e. in melanoma has averted futile surgery and unnecessary treatment costs (Figure 3) [2, 29]. The combined PET-CT over scored the standalone CT and PET in the re-staging tumor after years of free-disease survival whereby the distorted anatomy may not be easily distinguished from the site of tumor recurrent [29]. 18[F] FDG PET-CT has been shown to be useful for detection of nodal and distant metastases in patients with soft-tissue sarcomas compared with that at conventional imaging [30]

4.3. FDG PET-CT in tumor staging

The evaluation of tumor prior to any treatment or surgical intervention is vital as an inappropriate staging may lead to unnecessary treatment course and cost and futile surgery. Integrated molecular imaging technique offers a high accuracy in the staging of tumor especially those which are equivocal on the structural imaging (CT, MRI) as correlated on the clinical background. Metabolic information by PET is always the essential element in the determination of an altered metabolism preceding any structural change (Figure 4). There are many published data that support this evidence in many tumor streams. A retrospective analysis included 50 patients with 55 clinical events of elevated or increasing CEA level who underwent FDG PET-CT and MDCT for suspected tumor recurrence, FDG PET-CT has higher sensitivity than MDCT in the identification of sites of recurrent and metastatic disease in patients with colorectal cancer and an elevated CEA level [31]. In a study based on 172 non small cell lung carcinoma (NSCLC) patients from a prospective clinical study who underwent diagnostic, contrast-enhanced helical CT and integrated PET-CT on the treatment costs, the diagnostic effectiveness in terms of correct TNM staging was 40% (31/77) for CT alone and 60% (46/77) for PET-CT. For the assessment of resectability (tumor stages Ia-IIIa vs. IIIb-IV), 65 of 77 patients (84%) were staged correctly by PET-CT (CT alone, 70% [54/77]). The incremental cost-effectiveness ratios per correctly staged patient were $3,508 for PET-CT versus CT alone [32]. Data on 122 patients with PET-CT scans as part of their initial staging of lymphoma, PET-CT upstages 17% of cases and detects occult splenic involvement [33]

4.4. FDG PET-CT in predicting tumor aggressiveness

In addition, the degree of metabolic defect via semi quantitative analysis, standard uptake value (SUV) could predict tumor aggressiveness and the overall patient survival as high SUV values correlates with poor disease prognosis (Figure 5). Predicting tumor aggressiveness is

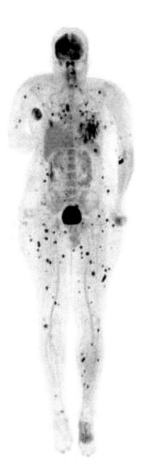

Figure 3. PET-CT restaging in 56-year-old man who had partial amputation of the right forearm for malignant melanoma. The MIP-PET image shows innumerable hypermetabolic foci of metastatic lesion throughout the body (subcentimetre lesions are imperceptible on the CT images; correlated CT image is not shown).

important as early decision on the management strategy of a patient suffering from an advance
tumor could lead to an improved prognosis. A particular type of tumor i.e. thymoma which
their cellular make-up does not always exhibit malignant entity when a clinical assessment is
equivocally ascertained, the role of molecular imaging employing PET with glucose analog
has been shown to impact the prognostic outcome in many instances [34]. In a retrospective
study by Lopei et al of 91 patients with follicular lymphoma (FL), end-treatment PET-CT in
FL has high accuracy and appears to be a good predictor of progression free survival (PFS)
and patient outcome, irrespective of grading [35]. Due to clonal heterogeneity in some tumors,
FDG-PET could potentially become a determinant factor in determining which cells types may
be aggressive or have de-differentiated. In a study of 23 patients with neuroendocrine tumor

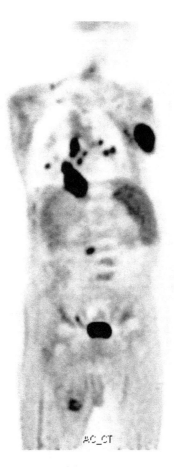

Figure 4. PET-CT Staging of recently diagnosed non-Hodgkin lymphoma by CT in 58-year-old woman. Coronal PET image shows involvement of the spleen (CT image was normal; correlated image is not shown) for which the disease was upstage to stage 3.

(NET), Fathinul et al suggested a cut-off value of 9.1 to predict tumor with an aggressive potential. This is in line with other study that suggests FDG-avid NET is usually more aggressive than FDG-negative lesions whereby the former may be benefited from systemic treatment (chemotherapy) [36]. In this regards, the role of molecular imaging is of prime important when structural changes are lacking of certain valuable information of the tumor altered cellular biology.

4.5. FDG PET-CT and the patient management

The use of PET-CT is potentially reported to change of the primary diagnosis in approximately 16% of cases, whereas PET-CT resulted in a change in staging and treatment plan in approximately 28% to 32% of the cases, respectively (Table 5) [37]. One area in which FDG PET can play a significant role is in establishing response to treatment [38]. Current procedures to monitor therapy use mainly anatomical imaging modalities, such as CT, even though metabolic changes in tumors may occur earlier than, or even instead of, anatomical size changes. A significant metabolic change can be established by comparing uptake values from pre- and post treatment scans, although such comparisons can only be made accurately on attenuation-corrected, quantitative PET images.

Patient (P)	Histological Diagnosis	AJCC (6th ed) Staging before PET-CT Scan	AJCC (6th ed) Staging after PET-CT Scan
P1	NPC	Stage III	Stage IVB
P2	NPC	Stage IVB	Stage IVB
P3	Ca larynx	Stage I	Stage I
P4	Sarcoma of tonsil	Stage II	
P5	Metastatic papillary carcinoma of thyroid	NA	Stage I
P6	Occult node-Metastatic carcinoma of neck	NA	FDG uptake only in Lymph nodes
P7	Primary adnexal Ca	Stage I	Stage I
P8	Ca larynx	Stage I	Stage I
P9	Thyroglossal cyst with focal papillary carcinoma	NA	Stage III
P10	NPC	Stage II	Stage IVA
P11	NPC	Stage I	Stage I
P12	NPC	Stage III	Stage IVA
P13	Ca tonsil	Stage IV	Stage IVB
P14	Lymphoma	Stage I	Stage III
P15	NPC	Stage I	Stage I
P16	Metastatic adenocarcinoma of base of skull	NA	Stage IVC
P17	Ca hard palate	Stage II	Stage IVC
P18	NPC	Stage III	Stage IVB
P19	NPC	Stage II	Stage IVC
P20	NPC	Stage II	Stage IVA
P21	NPC	Stage III	Stage IVC
P22	NPC	Stage III	Stage IVC
P23	NPC	Stage I	Stage IVC

Table 5. Data of 23 patients with head and neck tumors on the disease staging before and after the PET-CT evaluation (39)

5. FDG PET-CT as a predictor of overall patient survival

The use of FDG as a ligand in particular for a molecular imaging technique i.e. PET-CT has been shown to provide prognostic stratification. The complete metabolic response of tumor as imaged on the FDG-PET-CT scan implies a favourable change in tumor apoptosis which is correlated with good prognosis. In a study by Fathinul et al focusing on the esophageal tumor as group-staged by I–IIA and IIB–IV had a 1-year survival of 50% and 25% respectively [40]. Patient with size of primary tumor (<4.5cm) had significantly ($p< 0.036$) better survival than those with large size (>4.5cm). A SUV_{max} of > 5.5 in the primary tumor [Hazard Ratio (HR) 58.65; 95% confidence interval, p=0.032] and presence of FDG-avid lymph node (HR 20.83; $p =$ 0.010) were strongly predictive of poor overall survival on multivariate analysis Figure (5)

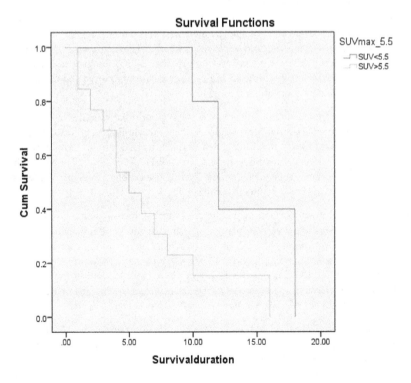

Figure 5. The survival prognostication of a cohort of 18 patients with esophageal cancers as stratified by the SUVmax cut-off of 5.5.

6. FDG-PET-CT in coronary artery disease

Cardiovascular disease is one of the leading causes of death. It carries great impact on the patients, their families as well as the country socially and financially. Cardiology is also a rapidly advancing field, with new approaches to prevention, risk stratification, diagnosis and treatment. Early detection and appropriate risk stratification will help to optimize resources and to ensure that appropriate treatment will be provided to those who would benefit from it. Diagnostic methods commonly used in the detection and risk stratification of coronary artery disease include exercise stress testing, stress echocardiography, multi-slice computed tomography, Single Photon Emission Computed Tomography (SPECT) and invasive coronary angiography. Each of these modalities has its own advantages, disadvantages and limitations.

The management of coronary artery disease includes lifestyle modifications, medications, percutaneous coronary interventions and coronary artery bypass surgery. Invasive procedures carries risks, as well as its associated costs, thus it is imperative that proper selection of patients are made based on the clinical presentation and the results of investigations. Positron Emission Tomography is a relatively new diagnostic modality with the potential to address some of the limitations of current commonly used diagnostic methods. Cardiology imaging using Integrated PET-CT equipment demonstrates an improved method in detecting abnormal coronary circulation. The resolution of PET-CT images are superior than SPECT imaging as a result of improved camera resolution and specification, high energy positron captured and CT attenuation corrected in all PET data acquisition.

In PET, 18F-FDG is the tracer most frequently used to assess myocardial viability (41-43). Since FDG is a glucose analogue, the substance is used to evaluate cardiac glucose utilization where mitochondria plays pivotal role in its utilization. The initial uptake in myocardial tissue is comparable to glucose uptake. After phosphorylation, 18F FDG-6-PO4 is trapped within cardiac tissues and the metabolism ends before the Krebs cycle enabling imaging due to the strong signal from radiation source emitted by 18-F isotope.

Evaluation of residual glucose metabolism, a hallmark of viable myocardium, by FDG –PET is considered the most sensitive non-invasive tool to assess the myocardial viability[44-45]. Viable myocardium shows preserved FDG uptake whereas, markedly reduced or absent uptake indicates scar tissue formation (Figure 6-7). Most studies relate myocardial perfusion to the FDG PET viability. FDG accumulates in the myocytes independent of the vascular enrichment. Therefore quantitative assessment of the FDG concentration in the myocardium is vital as it indicates viable tissue which is amenable to be reversed [46].

Integrated PET-CT system can be utilized in myocardial perfusion study using 82-Rubidium (Figure 8). The dynamic data acquisition during rest and stress are quantifiable using dedicated coronary flow quantification software (47-49). Abnormal readings will be obtained in coronary obstruction and endothelial dysfunction using this method. Myocardial flow reserve quantification has high sensitivity and positive predictive value in correlation with left ventricular function (Figure 9). Thus, can be recommended as a suitable non invasive tool in making clinical decision for managing patients with coronary artery disease

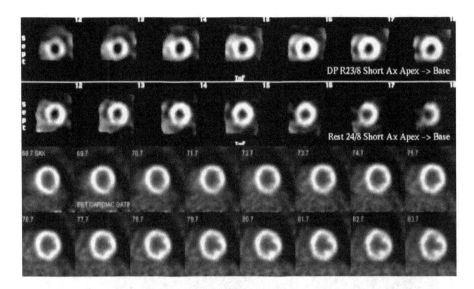

Figure 6. The transaxial non-gated static SPECT image (1st and 2nd rows from the top) and PET-CT image (3rd and 4th rows). There is a reversible defect seen affecting the posterior wall of left ventricle which filled up during FDG PET-CT study in keeping with a reversible ischaemic myocardial segment.

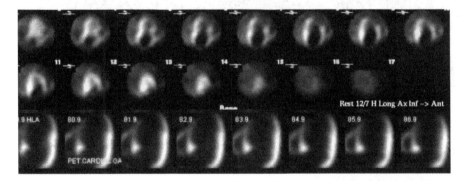

Figure 7. The horizontal long axis non-gated static SPECT image (1st and 2nd rows from the top) and PET-CT image (3rd row). There is an irreversible defect seen affecting the apex of left ventricle in keeping with an infarcted myocardial segment

7. FDG PET-CT in infection

FDG is a well known in-vivo biomarker indicating the rate of tissue metabolism. The initial course of direction for clinical utility of PET-CT in oncology is now widened into the field of infections [50-52]. Increase cancer tissue metabolism are thought to be related to raised in surrounding inflammatory reaction as demonstrated by Kubota resulting from high accumu-

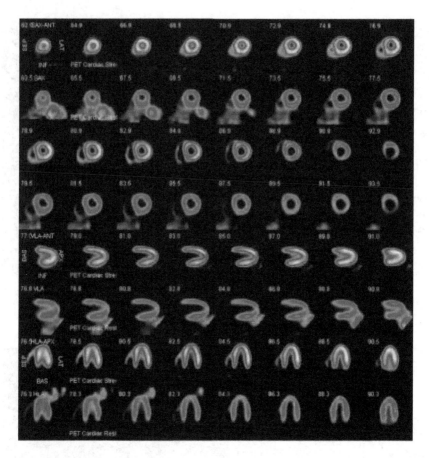

Figure 8. Myocardial perfusion 82-Rb demonstrating high quality images in a normal patient.

lation of macrophages and granulation tissues [53]. Likewise, in infection, initial increased in local hyperemia and capillary permeability will lead to aggregation of granulocytes, leucocytes and macrophage at the point of entry by pathogens. This cascade of events will lead to increased in local glucose consumption. The signals from annihilation process of positively charged beta particles emitted from radioactive fluorinated glucose molecules in-situ will be detected by PET camera during PET-CT imaging where the activity can be semi-quantified using the semi-quantitative uptake value (SUV). The SUV of infective foci are often raised above the background 18F-FDG soft tissue activity.

Despite their known clinical entity, the use of 18F-FDG PET-CT in establishing the diagnosis of infection and inflammatory condition is still controversial. A meta analysis conducted [54-62] from a series of review articles found that 18F-FDG demonstrate highest utility in cases of chronic osteomyelitis, hip prostheses, diabetic foot, fever of unknown origin, vasculitis,

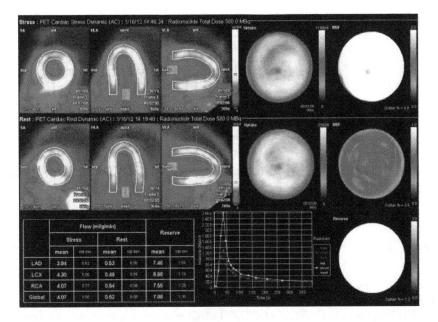

Figure 9. Quantification analysis of 82Rb Myocardial Perfusion PET CT study of a young man demonstrating normal global stress and rest flow. The coronary reserve is normal.

acquired immunodeficiency syndrome, and vascular graft infection. The role of CT during integrated PET CT imaging in the diagnosis of these conditions may range between CT for anatomical correlation and attenuation correction to non attenuation corrected fused images. In some condition, informations obtained from CT which may be classical and pathognomonic can be an important adjunct features in deciding clinical management.

For example, PET using ^{18}F-FDG appears to be a highly sensitive method in detecting infective foci in the bone. Histologically, the ^{18}F-FDG avidity defines the area of fibroblast proliferation and neovascularisation with mononuclear cell infiltration at the granulation tissue formation whereby these cells utilises most of their energy from the trapped ^{18}F-FDG for cells metabolism [63-65]FDG-PET is sensitive than the standalone CT in delineating evidence of implant infection (Figure 10)

However, since artefact through beam hardening effect of X-ray from CT scan during PET-CT study can significantly obscure the underlying pathology, often non attenuation corrected images are being the standard reference in making clinical decision for major interventional procedure. Thus, a combined PET-CT study can be a very useful modality in solving painful hip problem in a patient with hip prosthesis.

18F-FDG PET-CT can also be a useful technique in ruling out infection in critically ill patients under Intensive Care Unit (ICU) management. Study has shown that a normal scan exclude prolonged use of antibiotic in these patients [66]. Combined CT and PET have also been

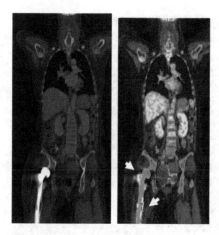

Figure 10. Coronal CT (left panel) is insensitive in delineating implant infection as the FDG PET-CT (right panel) is clearly showing increased FDG uptake along the implant denoting underlying infection (arrow heads).

reported to be useful in detecting vascular prosthesis infection. The presence of infection in such cases usually in elderly, will justify for removal of infected prosthesis. More recently, Rudd et al disclosed the capability of 18F-FDG-PET-CT in identifying and quantifying vascular inflammation within atherosclerotic plaques [67].These vulnerable plagues carry high risk of auto detachment causing embolisation and ischaemic infarct to vital organs increasing the risk for cerebral vascular accident and ischaemic heart disease (Figure 11). Positive correlation between FDG uptake measurements in the left anterior descending artery with high risk factors of coronary artery diseases has been established [68].

The scope of FDG PET-CT study is widest in cancer imaging leading to increasing application of this powerful modality into clinical practice. There has been significant evidence showing non exclusivity of FDG as a tumor marker observed with increase FDG uptake seen in a wide range of infection and inflammatory conditions[69]. Examples are chronic granulomatous infections like sarcoidoses, infections by tuberculosis, fungal infection like aspergillosis and narcoidoses which are known to demonstrate high FDG uptake. Although they can jeopardize the accuracy of integrated imaging interpretation in malignancy, their high standardized uptake value (SUV) during semiquantification on FDG PET-CT can be exploited and utilized as an important localizing tool for guided biopsy and potentially useful for navigating response to treatment [70].

8. FDG PET-CT in pre-clinical application

PET/SPECT neuroreceptor and metabolic imaging, as well as conventional and functional MR imaging, MR spectroscopy, optical imaging, and other techniques, is utilized almost routinely to help establish proof of- mechanism studies for new drugs, especially at the interface between

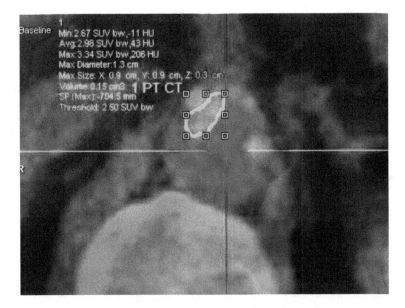

Figure 11. Cross sectional image of abdominal aorta demonstrating vulnerable plague at 11 o'clock (SUVmax of 3.3) and 3 o'clock position. The green and red cursors are shown to be crossing the centre of the aorta

preclinical and early phase 1 studies. In particular the use of FDG as a PET probe, its SUVmax values have been shown to correlate with histologic grade in heterogeneous series of bone and soft-tissue sarcomas [71]. The potential for molecular imaging in small animals to increase knowledge of drug effects in models of human cancer has been recognized around the world. This has been embraced as a means of decreasing the time taken to indentify agents that merit clinical trial and to decrease the cost of drug development [72]. The ability to extrapolate from animals to human studies makes PET a logical technique for both pre-clinical testing of new therapeutic drugs and for the validation of new tracers that might be relevant to the evaluation of human diseases. Manipulation of cells and tissues to produce animal models that mimic human diseases provides a useful system to test new tracers. At a pragmatic level, a short feedback loops between studies in mice and then in man is important. While unrestrained proliferation has been described as a hallmark of cancer and is a target of several targeted anti-cancer therapeutics, due to differences in blood thymidine levels and in the metabolism of PET probe which look at cell proliferation i.e. Fluorothymidine (FLT), both uptake and excretion of this tracer show significant differences in biodistribution in different species.

9. FDG PET-CT in non-clinical application

The development of imaging technologies, including hybrid systems allow the evaluation of gene expression in various cancers. The underlying original genetic problems of cancer can be monitored by PET using radiolabeled metabolic substances including glucose, amino acids or nucleotides. Sometimes, molecular imaging means genetic imaging or molecular-genetic imaging in which the assessment is based on the reporter genes and labeled antisense oligo-nucleotide probes [73].

Radiolabeled antisense oligonucleotide probes have been applied to image endogenous gene expression at the transcription level [74]. In diagnostic radiology, CT and ultrasonography (US) have been examined as means of molecular-genetic imaging. In PET, dopamine 2 receptor (D_2R) gene is used as an imaging reporter gene, because of the availability of the well established radiolabeled probe ^{18}F-fluoroethlspiperone (FESP) [75]. Moreover, Furukawa et al. [76] have designed a reporter gene imaging system based on ^{18}F-labeed estradiol and human estrogen receptor ligand (hERL) binding domain in access of various tissues for gene therapy monitoring.

Several researchers have investigated the use of γ-emitters for molecular imaging [77, 78]; examples include the somatostatin receptor (SSTr) 2 (SSTr2) gene and [111]Inoctreotide [79], the norepinephrine transporter gene and ^{131}I-labeled metaiodobenzylguanidine (^{131}I-MIBG) [80], sodium/iodide symporter (NIS) gene and radioiodines or ^{99m}Tc-pertechnetate [33, 34]. Jacobs et al. [81] demonstrated the first human PET image of HSV1-tk gene expression in a glioma patient.

10. Molecular imaging: Future perspective

Molecular imaging is now being accepted by many (physicians) as an important platform in translating genetic defect through aberrant protein function and cellular transformation and development. Nevertheless, the sensitivity of molecular imaging techniques is varied depend-ing on the type of radiopharmaceutical marker used in signaling the biological processes. In particular, the use of FDG as a ligand PET-CT has many limitations. The most obvious example of this is in the brain where high glucose utilisation by the normal cerebral cortex can mask brain tumors, particularly those of well differentiated. In addition, some tumors with high metastatic potential can have relatively low FDG-uptake. Similarly, the specificity of FDG–PET is also imperfect with some benign conditions, particularly granulomatous lesions i.e. tuberculosis, having high FDG uptake. These very real limitations of FDG used in the molec-ular imaging technique have enticed the search for alternative radiotracers which signal different biological disease process. Several alternative PET-radiopharmaceuticals are cur-rently being investigated, which have the potential to reveal the proliferation rate, oxygen utilization, drug resistance properties and the viability of the tumors. Examples of new PET tracers include fluoroethyltyrosine (FET) for brain tumor imaging; the proliferation marker 18F-fluorothymidine (FLT) to assess bone marrow reserves and the exploitation of dual tracer strategy i.e. FDG and 68 Ga DOTA –octreotate for staging and therapeutic response in neuroendocrine tumor would promise a more complete assessment of disease process and tumor biology. The choline analogue 18F-fluorocholine (FCH) for patients with rising prostate specific antigen levels would potentially have an impact on the management strategy and thus improve the overall patient survival. It is likely that the continuing success of molecular imaging will rest on the future development of more disease specific ligand or tracer, used in specific combination to answer the important clinical question.

Acknowledgements

This work was supported by the Pusat Pengimejan Diagnostik Nuklear, Universiti Putra Malaysia.

Author details

Fathinul Fikri Ahmad Saad[1*], Abdul Jalil Nordin[1], Hishar Hassan[1], Cheah Yoke Kqueen[2] and W.F.E Lau[3]

*Address all correspondence to: ahmadsaadff@gmail.com

1 Centre for Diagnostic Nuclear imaging, University Putra Malaysia, Serdang, Selangor, Malaysia

2 Biomedicine Unit Faculty of Medicine and Health Science, University Putra Malaysia, Serdang, Selangor, Malaysia

3 Department of Radiology, the University of Melbourne, Centre for Molecular Imaging, The Peter MacCallum, Cancer Centre, Australia

References

[1] Mankoff D. A definition of molecular imaging. Breast Cancer Res. 2008; 10(Suppl 1): S3.

[2] Niikura N, Costelloe CM, Madewell JE, Hayashi N, Yu TK, Liu J, Palla SL, Tokuda Y, Theriault RL, Hortobagyi GN, Ueno NT. FDG-PET-CT compared with conventional imaging in the detection of distant metastases of primary breast cancer. Oncologist. 2011;16(8):1111-9.

[3] Kim SK, Allen-Auerbach M, Goldin J, Fueger BJ, Dahlbom M, Brown M, Czernin J, Schiepers C. Accuracy of PET-CT in characterization of solitary pulmonary lesions. J Nucl Med. 2007 ;48(2):214-20.

[4] Pim A.J , Henriette M. Quarles van U ,Henk-Jan B, Marie J. H , Shulamiet H. W, Lor-entz G. Q and John M. K . CT and ^{18}F-FDG PET for Noninvasive Detection of Splenic Involvement in Patients with Malignant Lymphoma.. AJR 2009. 192 (3): 745-753

[5] Ozkan E, Soydal C, Araz M, Kir KM, Ibis E. The role of 18F-FDG PET-CT in detecting colorectal cancer recurrence in patients with elevated CEA levels. Nucl Med Com-mun. 2012 ;33(4):395-402.

[6] Tel-Pogossian MM, Phleps ME, Hoffman EJ, Mullani NA. A positron emission trans-axial tomography for nuclear imaging (PET), Radiology 1975, 114(1):89-98

[7] Bonekamp D, Hammoud DA, Pomper MG, Molecular imaging, techniques and cur-rent clinical applications. Applied Radiology. 2010 May; 39(5); 10-21

[8] Silver S . U.S. Food and Drug Administration. Ultrasound imaging; 2012 . http://www.fda.gov/RadiationEmittingProducts/RadiationEmittingProductsandProce-dures/MedicalImaging/ucm115357.htm (accessed 3 August 2012)

[9] Martin GP, Henry FV, Carolyn JA. what is molecular imaging;?. SNM Molecular Imaging Centre of Excellence http://www.molecularimagingcenter.org/img/mi_post-er/What_is_MI_Poster.pdf (accessed 3 August 2012)

[10] Hornak JP. The basic of MRI .http://www.cis.rit.edu/htbooks/mri/chap-1/chap-1.htm (accessed 3 August 2012)

[11] Shiel WC. Magnetic resonance imaging .http://www.medicinenet.com/mri_scan/arti-cle.htm#1whatis (accessed 3 August 2012)

[12] Gambhir SS. SNM Molecular Imaging Centre of Excellence. Just what is molecular imaging; 2007 http://www.molecularimagingcenter.org/index.cfm?PageID=8594 (ac-cessed 3 August 2012)

[13] Wood KA, Hoskin PJ, Saunders MI. Positron emission tomography in oncology: a re-view. Clinical Oncology. 2007; 19: 237-255

[14] Marcian E. VD, Alnawaz R, and Brian D. R. PET and SPECT Imaging of Tumor Biol-ogy: New Approaches towards Oncology Drug Discovery and Development. Curr Comput Aided Drug Des. 2008; 4(1): 46–53.

[15] Gambhir SS, Czermin J, Schwimmer J, Silverman DH, Coleman RE, Phelps ME. A tabulated summary of the FDG PET literature. Journal of Nuclear Medicine. 2001; 42: 1S-93S

[16] Arman R, Habib Z. PET versus SPECT: strengths, limitations and challenges. Nuclear Medicine Communications 2008, Vol 29 No 3

[17] Kim CK, Gupta NC, Chandramouli B, Alavi A. Standardized uptake values of FDG: body surface area correction is preferable to body weight correction. J Nucl Med. 1994. 35: 164-167

[18] Matthew D. T, Philip W.S, William K.B., Mark R.W, Nicholas T, Brian R. S., Benjamin D. K., Christine L. L. , David R. J.. Fluorodeoxyglucose positron emission tomography and tumor marker expression in non–small cell lung cancer. *J Thorac Cardiovasc Surg.* 2009. 137, 43-48

[19] International Commission on Radiological Protection. ICRP publication Oxford, England: Pergamon, 1991; 60.

[20] Guillet B, Quentin P, Waultier S. Technologist radiation exposure in routine clinical practice with ^{18}F-FDG PET. Journal of Nuclear Medicine Technology. 2005; 33(3): 175-179.

[21] Tracy A. J, Terry T. Y, Greta T. Radiation Dose for Body CT Protocols: Variability of Scanners at One Institution. AJR: 2009 193:1141–1147

[22] Zito F, Luca Z, Cristina C. Radiation exposure during PET-CT transmission imaging with 6 and 64-slice-CT scanners. J Nucl Med. 2009; 50 (Supplement 2):1485

[23] Buck AK, Hermann K, Stargardt T, Dechow T, Krause BJ, Schreyyogg J: Econoevaluation of PET and PET-Ct in oncology: Evidence and Methodologic Approaches. J Nucl Med 2010, 51 (3): 401-412.].

[24] Warburg O. The Metabolism of Tumors. London, U.K.: Arnold Constable; 1930.

[25] Kroemer G, Pouyssegur J. Tumor cell metabolism: cancer's Achilles' heel. Cancer Cell. 2008;13:472–482.

[26] Bayani J, Selvarajah S, Maire G, Vukovicc B, Al-Romaihd K, Zielenska M, et al. Genomic mechanisms and measurement of structural and numerical instability in cancer cells. Semin Cancer Biol. Feb 2007;17(1):5-18.

[27] Yon M S, Kyung S L, Byung T K, et al. 18F-FDG PET-CT of Thymic Epithelial Tumors: Usefulness for Distinguishing and Staging Tumor Subgroups. J Nucl Med 2006; 47:1628–1634

[28] Pottgen C, Levegrun S, Theegarten D, et al. Value of 18 F-fluoro-2-deoxy-glucose-positron emission tomography/computed tomography in non-small-cell lung cancer for prediction of pathologic response and times to relapse after neoadjuvant chemoradiotherapy. Clin Cancer Res. 2006; 12:97–106

[29] Eubank WB, Mankoff DA, Schmiedl UP, et al. Imaging of oncologic patients: benefits of combined CT and FDG PET in the diagnosis of malignancy. AJR Am J Roentgenol 1998; 171:1103-1110.

[30] Johnson GR, Zhuang H, Khan J. Role of positron emission tomography with fluorine-18-deoxyglucose in the detection of local recurrent and distant metastatic sarcoma. Clin Nucl Med 2003;28:815–820.

[31] Metser U, You J, McSweeney S, Freeman M, Hendler A. Assessment of tumor recurrence in patients with colorectal cancer and elevated carcinoembryonic antigen level:

FDG PET-CT versus contrast-enhanced 64-MDCT of the chest and abdomen.AJR Am J Roentgenol. 2010 Mar;194(3):766-71.

[32] Schreyögg J, Weller J, Stargardt T, Herrmann K, Bluemel C, Dechow T, Glatting G, Krause BJ, Mottaghy F, Reske SN, Buck AK. Cost-effectiveness of hybrid PET-CT for staging of non-small cell lung cancer. J Nucl Med. 2010 Nov;51(11):1668-75.

[33] Ngeow J. Y. Y. , Quek R. H. H. , Ng D. C. E. , Hee S. W. , Tao M. , Lim L. C. , Tan Y. H. and Lim S. T. High SUV uptake on FDG–PET-CT predicts for an aggressive B-cell lymphoma in a prospective study of primary FDG–PET-CT staging in lymphoma. Oxford Journals Medicine Annals of Oncology.20(9): 1543-154

[34] Yon, M S., Kyung, S L., Byung, T K. 18F-FDG PET-CT of Thymic Epithelial Tumors: Usefulness for Distinguishing and Staging Tumor Subgroups. J Nucl Med; 2006. 47:1628–1634

[35] Lopci E, Zanoni L, Chiti A, Fonti C, Santi I, Zinzani PL, Fanti S. FDG PET-CT predictive role in follicular lymphoma. Eur J Nucl Med Mol Imaging. 2012 May;39(5): 864-71.

[36] 36 Fathinul F., Nordin A. J., Zanariah H., Kroiss A., Uprimny C., Donnemiller E., Kendler D., Virgolini I. J. (2011). Localisation and prediction of recurrent phaechromocytoma/paraganglioma (PCC/PGL) using diagnostic 18[F] FDG PET-CT. Cancer Imaging, 3(11), Spec No A: S114-S115

[37] Kruser TJ, Bradley KA, Bentzen SM, et al. The impact of hybrid PET-CT scan on overall oncologic management, with a focus on radiotherapy planning: a prospective, blinded study. Technol Cancer Res Treat. 2009;8(2):149-58.

[38] Pottgen C, Levegrun S, Theegarten D. Value of 18 F-fluoro-2-deoxy-Dglucose-positron emission tomography/computed tomography in non-small-cell lung cancer for prediction of pathologic response and times to relapse after neoadjuvant chemoradiotherapy. Clin Cancer Res. 2006. 12:97–106

[39] Fathinul, F., Subha, S.T. Azman, M ., Nordin. AJ. Clinical applications of the standard uptake values of the contrasted 18[F]-FDGPET-CT in nasopharyngeal carcinoma patients Cancer Imaging . 2011. 11: 40 .DOI: 10.1102/1470-7330.2011.9049.

[40] F Fathinul , AJ Nordin, R Dharmendran, P Vikneswaran . The value of pretreatment PET-CT in predicting survival in patient with esophageal cancer. Proceeding at the International Cancer Imaging Society Meeting and 12th Annual Teaching Course; ICIS 2012, 4-6 October 2-012, Oxford, United Kingdom

[41] Andreas H. Mahnken, Ralf Koos, Marcus Katoh, Joachim E. W, Elmar S, Arno B, Rolf W. G, Harald P. K , Assessment of Myocardial Viability in Reperfused Acute Myocardial Infarction Using 16-Slice Computed Tomography in Comparison to Magnetic Resonance Imaging. JACC .2005.45(12):2042–7

[42] Ichiro M, Junichi T, Kenichi N, Norihisa T and Kinichi H. Myocardial viability assess-
      ment using nuclear imaging. Annals of Nuclear Medicine 2003; 17(3).169–179

[43] Katherine C. W and Joao A.C. L. Developments Noninvasive Imaging of Myocardial
      Viability: Current Techniques and Future . Circ. Res . 2003;93;1146-1158

[44] PET-CT: Challenge for Nuclear Cardiology. Markus S, Sibylle Z, and Stephan G. N . J
      Nucl Med 2005; 46:1664 –1678

[45] Harald P. K et al. Assessment of reversible myocardial dysfunction in chronic ischae-
      mic heart disease: comparison of contrast- enhanced cardiovascular magnetic reso-
      nance and a combined positron emission tomography–single photon emission
      computed tomography imaging protocol . European Heart Journal (2006) 27, 846–853

[46] Antti S, Heikki U, Sami K, Juhani K. Integrated anatomy and viability assessment
      PET-CT. Euro Intervention Supplement 2010. (6), Supplmnt (G); 132-137

[47] Parkash R et al ; Potential utility of rubidium 82 PET quantification in patients with 3-
      vessel coronary artery disease. Journal of Nuclear Cardiology 441 (1) 4;440-49

[48] Mario P, Andrea S, Giovanni S, Alberto C .Assessment of coronary flow reserve using
      single photon emission computed tomography with technetium 99m–labeled trac-
      ers . J Nucl Cardiol 2008;15:456-65

[49] Gilbert J. Zoghbi, Todd A. Dorfman, Ami E. Iskandrian, The Effects of Medications
      on Myocardial Perfusion. Journal of the American College of Cardiology. 2008. 52(6).

[50] Chantal P. BR, Elisabeth M. H. A. deK, FransH. M. C, JosW. M. van derM, WimJ. G.
      O. Clinical value of FDG PET in patients with fever of unknown origin and patients
      suspected of focal infection or inflammation. Eur J Nucl Med Mol Imaging .2004.
      31:29–37

[51] Patz E. F., Lowe V. J., Hoffman J. M., Paine S. S., Burrowes P., Coleman R.E.. Focal
      Pulmonary Abnormalities: Evaluation with F-18 Fluorodeoxyglucose PET Scanning.
      Radiology 1993, 188, 487-490.

[52] Alessio I, Laure F, Nicolas L, Jean-JB,Francis P, ,O Romain K, Yves H, Emmanuel A,
      Andre' CF-18 FDG PET-CT as a Valuable Imaging Tool for Assessing Treatment Effi-
      cacy in Inflammatory and Infectious Diseases. Clin Nucl Med 2010;35: 86 –90.

[53] Kubota R., Yamada S., Kamada K., Ishiwata K., Tamahashi N., Tatsuo, I.Intratumoral
      Distribution of Fluorine-18 Fluorodeoxyglucose In Vivo: High Accumulation in Mac-
      rophages and Granulation Tissues Studied by Microautoradiography. J. Nucl. Med.
      1992, 33, 1972-1980.

[54] Stumpke KD, Dazzi H, Schaffner A et al. Infection imaging using whole-body FDG-
      PET. Eur J Nucl Med .2000. 27:822–832

[55] Zhuang H, Alavi A .18-Fluorodeoxyglucose positron emission tomographic imaging in the detection and monitoring of infection and inflammation. Semin Nucl Med 2002. 32:47–59

[56] Chacko TK, Zhuang H, Nakhoda KZ . Applications of fluorodeoxyglucose positron emission tomography in the diagnosis of infection. Nucl Med Commun 2003. 24:615–624

[57] Love C, Tomas MB, Tronco GG et al. FDG PET of infection and inflammation. Radiographics .2005. 25:1357–1368

[58] Stroebel K, Stumpe KDM . PET-CT in musculoskeletal infection. Semin Musculoskelet Radiol. 2007. 11:353–364

[59] Basu S, Chryssikos BA, Moghadam-Kia S et al . Positron emission tomography as a diagnostic tool in infection: present role and future possibilities. Semin Nucl Med . 2009.39:36–51

[60] Petruzzi N, Shanthly N, Thakur M et al. Recent trends in soft tissue infection imaging. Semin Nucl Med 39.2009):115–123

[61] Glaudemans AWJM, Signore A . FDG-PET-CT in infections: the imaging method of choice? Eur J Nucl Med Mol Imaging . 2010. 37:1986–1991

[62] Marguerite T. Parisi . Functional imaging of infection: conventional nuclear medicine agents and the expanding role of 18-F-FDG PET . Pediatr Radiol .2011. 41:803–810

[63] Fathinul F, Nordin AJ. 18F-FDG PET-CT as a potential valuable adjunct to MRI in characterising the Brodie's abscess. Biomed Imaging Interv J 2010; 6(3):e26.

[64] Zhuang H, Alavi A. 18-fluorodeoxyglucose positron emission tomographic imaging in the detection and monitoring of infection and inflammation. Semin Nucl Med 2002;32(1):47–59.

[65] Yamada S, Kubota K, Ishiwata K et al . Intratumoral distribution of fluorine-18-fluorodeoxyglucose in vivo: high accumulation in macrophages and granulation tissues studied by microautoradiography. J Nucl Med 1992;33(11): 1972–1980.

[66] Koen S. S, Peter P, Chantal P. B.R, Wim J. G. O , Johannes G. van der H. F-18-fluorodeoxyglucose positron emission tomography combined with CT in critically ill patients with suspected infection. Intensive Care Med.2010. 36:504–511

[67] Rudd JH, Warburton EA, Fryer TD, et al. Imaging atherosclerotic plaque inflammation with [18F]-fluorodeoxyglucose positron emission tomography. Circulation 2002. 105:2708 –11

[68] Tobias S, Axel R, Sarah W, Konstantin Ni, Carsten R, Martin G, Paul C, Alexander B, Stefan F, Maximilian F. R, Peter B, Marcus H. Association of inflammation of the left anterior descending coronary artery with cardiovascular risk factors, plaque burden

and pericardial fat volume: a PET-CT study. Eur J Nucl Med Mol Imaging .2010. 37:1203–1212

[69] Basu S. Kumar, Alavi Abbas. PET and PET-CT imaging in infection and inflamma-tion: Its critical role in assessing complications related to therapeutic interventions in patients with cancer. Indian Journal of Cancer . 2010. 47 ; 4:371-379

[70] Nordin AJ, Noraini AR, Zaid FA , Popescu C. E.Cabrini G, Minniti L, Gay E, Rossetti C. Imaging pulmonary aspergillosis using 18F-Flourodeoxy -glucose biomarker in Positron Emission Tomography Computed Tomography. Proceedings of the World Medical Conference 2011. North Atlantic Universities Network

[71] Bastiaannet E, Groen H, Jager PL, et al. The value of FDG-PET in the detection, grad-ing and response to therapy of soft tissue and bone sarcomas: a systematic review and meta-analysis. Cancer Treat Rev 2004;30: 83–101

[72] Solomon B, Mc arthur G, Cullinace C, Zalcberg J, J, Hicks R. applications of positron emission tomography un the development of molecular targeted cancer therapeutics. BioDrugs. 2003: 17(5): 339-354

[73] Hyun, KJ., C, JK. Molecular-Genetic Imaging Based on Reporter Gene Expression. J Nucl Med. 2008; 49(6): 164-179

[74] Iyer, M, Sato, M, Johnson, M. Applications of molecular imaging in cancer therapy. Curr Gene Ther. 2005.;5:607–618

[75] MacLaren, DC., Gambhir, SS., Satyamurthy, N. Repetitive, noninvasive imaging of the dopamine D2 receptor as a reporter gene in living animals. Gene Ther. 1999;5:785–791

[76] Furukawa, T., Lohith, TG., Takamatsu, S. Potential of the FES-hERL PET reporter gene system: basic evaluation for gene therapy monitoring. Nucl Med Biol. 2006.;33:145–151

[77] Rogers, BE., Zinn, KR., Buchsbaum, DJ. Gene transfer strategies for improving radio-labeled peptide imaging and therapy. Q J Nucl Med. 2000.;44: 208–223.

[78] Haberkorn, U., Altmann, A, Mier, W., Eisenhut, M. Impact of functional genomics and proteomics on radionuclide imaging. Semin Nucl Med. 2004.;34:4–22.

[79] Rogers, BE., McLean, SF., Kirkman, RL. In vivo localization of [111In]- DTPA-D-Phe1-octreotide to human ovarian tumor xenografts induced to express the somatos-tatin receptor subtype 2 using an adenoviral vector. Clin Cancer Res. 1999.;5:383–393.

[80] Altmann, A., Kissel, M., Zitzmann, S. Increased MIBG uptake after transfer of the hu-man norepinephrine transporter gene in rat hepatoma.. J Nucl Med. 2003;44:973–980.

[81] Jacobs, A., Voges, J., Reszka, R.Positron-emission tomography of vectormediated gene expression in gene therapy for gliomas. Lancet.; 2001. 9283:727– 729.

Development of Articulation Simulation System Using Vocal Tract Model

Y.I. Sumita, K. Inohara, R. Sakurai, M. Hattori, S. Ino,
T. Ifukube and H. Taniguchi

Additional information is available at the end of the chapter

1. Introduction

During prosthetic treatment, dentists need to consider various factors, such as esthetics, speech, mastication, and swallowing, etc. Among them, the effect of prosthetic treatment on speech is an important concern for patients; thus, dentists must take care to avoid causing speech impairments during prosthodontic treatment, such as removable-type prostheses; partial or complete dentures and fixed-type prostheses; bridges and crowns. Since teeth and alveolar bone, maxillary bone are the main speech articulators, speech can be impaired by dental disorders such as missing teeth or the presence of insufficient prostheses.

Speech, masticatory, and swallowing disorders may occur in patients after the surgical resection of tumors with the head-and-neck region. Particularly, when a maxillary defect remains due to the extent of tumor resection, the nasal cavity constantly communicates with the vocal tract composed of the larynx, pharynx, and oral cavity and maxillectomy defect changes the vocal tract shape, inducing marked speech disorder. Concretely, communication between the nasal and oral cavities cannot be blocked, and breath passes through the nose and it causes hypernasality, resulting in unclear phonation. Acoustically, the relationship between the first and second formants of vowels alters [1].

However, the details have not yet been clarified. The production of vowels, an important element of voice, depend on the vocal tract shape [2]. In the source-filter theory [3], searching for the cause of speech disorder is considered possible based on the transfer characteristics in the vocal tract, which is a resonant tube, determined by measuring changes in the shape.

Maxillofacial prosthetic treatment such as the use of obturators is useful for rehabilitating the speech of maxillectomy patients as prostheses can be used to reconstruct maxillofacial defects

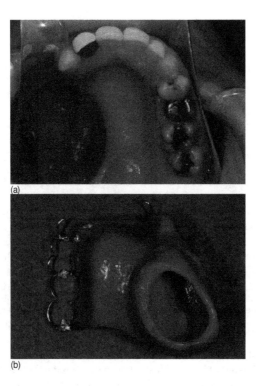

Figure 1. Dento-maxillary prosthesis for maxillectomy. Dento-maxillary prosthesis involves obuturator separate between nasal part and oral part. It prevent the air leakage and works well to improve the functional impairments.

including missing maxillary and alveolar bone and teeth. However, maxillofacial prosthetic treatment often takes a long time, as the prosthesis has to be adjusted until the optimal form has been achieved. This is particularly difficult because maxillofacial defects often have complicated structures, and patients sometimes suffer pain in the defect area and/or trismus Thus, a treatment protocol for maxillecyomys that is easy to apply and does not place an unnecessary burden on patients or doctors is required. Surgeons sometimes take CT images and MRI images of their patients to check for the presence of recurrent lesions, and we believe that CT images and MRI images could be useful for establishing an appropriate prosthetic treatment strategy for maxillectomy patients.

For example, if CT images and MRI images could be used to produce a speech simulation system, it would make it easier to design prostheses with optimal forms and reduce the time spent adjusting them.

The goal of our study is to make a vocal cord model from digital data and then use it to establish a speech simulation system for maxillofacial prosthetics and for the preliminary survey,in this study, we utilized an MRI images acquired while the subject phonated the sound /a/. The image was produced by the Advanced Telecommunications Research Institute International (ATR) Innovative Technology for Human Communication and published by the National Institute of Information and Communications Technology (NICT). Using this image, we prepared a phonating vocal tract model and confirmed the acoustic features with the acoustic analysis.

2. Materials and methods

2.1. Preparation of the vocal tract model

The "MRI database of Japanese vowel production" was used according to a licensing agreement with ATR-Promotions. The database contains MR images (in the DICOM format) that were acquired while a subject utter 5 vowels. We subjected the MRI image acquired while the subject uttered the sound /a/ to binarization in order to add tissue to our model using the software Mimics 11.11 (Materialise), according to the method reported by Inohara et al. [4,5] Dentition image data from the "MRI database of Japanese vowel production" were subsequently added to the image, and the vocal tract was extracted. The data were converted to the STL format and used to produce a solid mold with a Z406 3D printer system (Z Corp.).

First, the region to be molded was selected and simulated. Since teeth are not visualized by MRI, a toothless model was initially prepared despite the binarization method being employed, as shown in the right figure of Fig.2, and the dentition was subsequently added. Of the images published by ATR-Promotions, an image acquired while the subject held blueberry jam in their mouth was adopted since blueberry jam exhibitsed a contrast medium-like effect, and the teeth was visualized as transparent regions. Slices corresponding to the teeth were individually extracted, and image data (Fig.3) for the dentition alone were prepared.

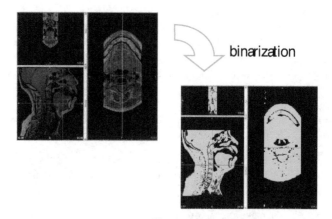

Figure 2. Binarization was applied to the image acquired while phonating/a/ using Mimics 111.11 following the method reported by Inohara et al.

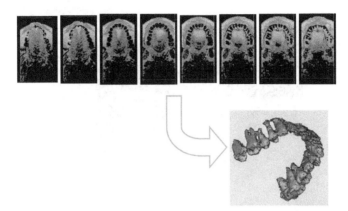

Figure 3. Tooth-extracted mold was prepared Of the images published by ATR-Promotions, the image acquired while holding blueberry jam in the mouth was adopted. Slices corresponding to the teeth were individually extracted, and obtained image data.

The prepared dentition image data were arranged at anatomically appropriate sites on the original image. Fig.4 shows the maxillary region after the dentition data had been added. The mandibular region also had dentition data added to it.

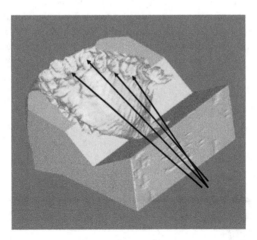

Figure 4. Maxillary region combined with dentition data The prepared dentition image data were arranged at anatomically appropriate sites on the original data to combine the images. Arrows: combined dentition data

These images were converted to the STL format and used to produce solid molds with the Z406 3D printer system at the Tsukuba Center of the National Institute of Industrial Science and Technology.

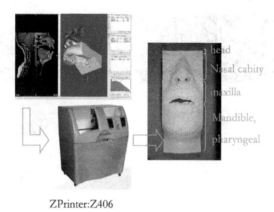

ZPrinter:Z406

Figure 5. Three-dimensional model was fabricated using ZPrinter. The model was separated 4 parts: head, nasal cabity, maxilla, mandible and pharyngteal.

2.2. Acoustic analysis

The completed vocal tract plaster models were combined, and an artificial larynx (Yourtone, Densei Inc.) was attached to the region corresponding to the vocal folds. In this preliminary study, a maxillary region with no defects was built. The initial maxillary region model had no defects, which was used to represent the preoperative conditions. Phonations were recorded for a model in a soundproof chamber. A microphone (Shure SM58) was placed 10 cm from the lips, and the sounds were recorded using a CSL4400 Computerized Speech Lab (Kay Pentax) and analyzed using the Wave Surfer software (KTH version 1.8.5) and the fast Fourier transform.

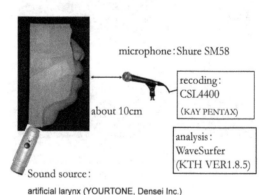

Figure 6. Acoustic analysis An artificial larynx (YOURTONE, Densei Inc.) was attached to the region corresponding to the vocal cords. A microphone was placed at a site 10cm from lips.

3. Result

When a model was present, the first (F1) and second (F2) formants were observed at 613 and 1,109 Hz, respectively, and no antiformant was present. The formants produced by the model deviated from those in the original recording by 8.6% for F1 and 6.0% for F2.

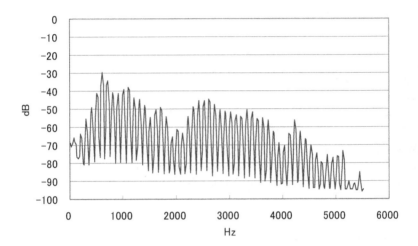

Figure 7. The data from 3D model

4. Discussion

We prepared a 3-dimensional model based on MRI data obtained from the "MRI database of Japanese vowel production" published by ATR-Promotions. We used binarization to add tissue data to an MRI image acquired during the phonation of the sound /a/ using the software Mimics 11.11 (Materialise), according to the method reported by Inohara et al. After adding dentition data to the image, we used the resultant image to produce a solid mold that simulated a vocal tract that was in constant communication with the nasal cavity. We then produced without maxillary defects which is simulated the preoperative condition for the preliminary survey in our research. In the model and added an artificial larynx to the region corresponding to the vocal folds.

However, we adopted an artificial larynx as the sound source, and its acoustic characteristics obviously influenced those of the model. Thus, it is necessary to accurately investigate the acoustic characteristics of the model by improving the measurement conditions, such as utilizing white noise.

Moreover, the formants produced by the model deviated from those of the original recording; i.e., by less than 10%, but these deviations are relatively small according to a study by Takemoto et al [6]. Our use of a model with a rigid body and the loss of sound through the boundaries between the constituent parts of the model were considered to have caused these differences.

The model was divided into 4 separately molded parts in order to allow us to produce defects that simulated various surgical conditions for our further study, which simulate the presence of maxillary defect, but it might be necessary to improve the position of the joins in the model and how they were held together.

For our further study, we would like to fabricate the models with maxilla defect which is simulated the maxillectomy and confirm the acoustic characteristics in order to establish the simulation system for maxillectomy patients. By making larger defects and/or changing the defect site, our model could be used to investigate the relationship between changes in the vocal tract and its transfer characteristics. It might also be possible to identify defect sites that cause antiformants to be produced.

Such investigations might allow potential speech disorders to be predicted before surgery, the modification of resection and/or reconstruction methods to avoid such problems, and the rapid production of optimally shaped prosthetics for filling surgical defects.

5. Conclusion

From the MRI image, it is possible to make the vocal tract model and its acoustic characteristics are confirmed with acoustic analysis

All study-related procedures and tests were approved by the Ethics Committee of Tokyo Medical and Dental University (Approval No. 166). 269

The MRI image were obtained from the "MRI database of Japanese vowel production", which was constructed during research commissioned by the National Institute of Information and Communications Technology: 'Research and development of human information communication' and performed and published by the ATR Innovative Technology for Human Communication. The obtained data were used and published based on a licensing agreement with ATR-Promotions.

The solid model was prepared with technical cooperation from Juri Yamashita and Kazumi Fukawa at the Tsukuba Center of the National Institute of Advanced Industrial Science and Technology.

This study was partially supported by a Grant-in-Aid for Young Scientists (B) from the Ministry of Education, Culture, Sports, Science and Technology, Japan.

This study was also supported by research grants from Support for Women Researchers from Tokyo Medical and Dental University.

Author details

Y.I. Sumita[1], K. Inohara[1,2], R. Sakurai[3], M. Hattori[1*], S. Ino[4], T. Ifukube[5] and H. Taniguchi[1]

*Address all correspondence to: sasamfp@tmd.ac.jp

1 Department of Maxillofacial Prosthetics, Graduate School, Tokyo Medical and Dental University, Japan

2 Keishu-kai Inohara Dental Clinic, Japan

3 Shinjuku-nishiguchi Dental Clinic, Japan

4 Human Technology Research Institute, National Institute of Advanced Industrial Science and Technology, Japan

5 Institute of Gerontology,The University of Tokyo, Japan

References

[1] Chiba, T, & Kajiyama, M. The Vowel, Its Nature and Structure; Tokyo-Kaiseikan ((1942).

[2] Sumita, Y. I, Ozawa, S, Mukohyama, H, Ueno, T, & Ohyama, T. Taniguchi H:Digital acoustic analysis of five vowels in maxillectomy patients. J Oral Rehabil((2002).

[3] Stevens, K. N. Acoustic Phonetics, MIT Press ((1998).

[4] Inohara, K, Sumita, Y. I, Ohbayashi, N, Ino, S, Kurabayashi, T, Ifukube, T, & Taniguchi, H. Standardization of thresholding for binary conversion of vocal tract modeling in Computed Tomography. J Voice,(2010).

[5] Ken Inohara, Yuka I. Sumita and Shuichi Ino ((2012). Extraction of Airway in Computed Tomography, Computed Tomography- Clinical Applications, Luca Saba (Ed.), 978-9-53307-378-1InTech, Available from: http://www.intechopen.com/books/computed-tomography-clinical-applications/extraction-of-airway-in-computed-tomography

[6] Takemoto, H, Mokhtari, P, & Kitamura, T. Acoustic analysis of the vocal tract during vowel production by finite-difference time-domain method," Journal of the Acoustical Society of America. 128 (6), (2010). , 3724-3738.

Chapter 4

MEDIMED Shared Regional PACS Center — Case Study

Karel Slavicek, Michal Javornik and Otto Dostal

Additional information is available at the end of the chapter

1. Introduction

Today most hospitals use PACS systems locally to store and evaluate picture data produced by various modalities (i.e. x-ray, ultrasound, computer tomography, etc.).

Outsourcing of archiving and communication technology offers a place for cooperation among hospitals and for utilization of the existing multimedia data on patients. This approach changes the thinking of medical specialists and teaches them to cooperate and share data on patients.

Gradually, it changes the thinking of medical specialists and gets them to cooperate and share data about patients in electronic form. It builds a network of medical specialists. The impact of this project is not only in patient care but also in the education of medical specialists. Some data (e.g. typical cases of given disease) stored in the MeDiMed PACS archive can be anonymized (i.e. personal data of patients is replaced by fictitious data) and used for educational purposes.

In the following chapters we briefly recall basic principles of the PACS and introduce the MeDiMed project.

1.1. PACS

The PACS (Picture Archiving and Communications System) is a currently used procedure and methodology for processing medical multimedia data obtained from picture acquisition machines like x-ray, ultrasound or computer tomography. Medicine picture data obtained from these machines (in PACS terminology called modalities) are stored in central PACS server. The PACS server then provides these multimedia data to viewing stations. Viewing stations serve for the radiologists to analyze and evaluate the multimedia data. This approach offers much more capabilities than former film medium. Viewing stations allow image transformation, combination of images from more modalities etc. National Electrical Manufacturers Association (NEMA) has developed a standard for communications between modalities, PACS servers and viewing stations. This standards is DICOM [3]. Currently DICOM version 3.0 is used in mostly all modalities and PACS servers. The structure of PACS is cleanly presented on the Figure 1.

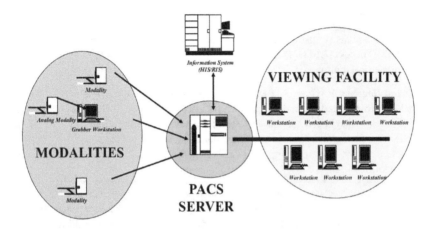

Figure 1. Common structure of PACS system. Modalities serve for acquisition of medicine multimedia data. These data are stored in PACS server and examined and analysed in viewing stations.

The digital processing of medicine multimedia data is very cost effective comparing to the legacy film based approach. A good example is the price comparison between a teleconsultation and a scenario where a doctor has to drive to visit a patient. The advantages of the telemedicine activities compared to the traditional methods are as follows:

• sharing of images among the cooperating institutions and their departments;

• cooperation with foreign medical partners;

• external long-term archiving of image data;

• management of other information associated and processed with image data;

• cost-benefit analysis performed by radiologists on standby duty at home;

• possibilities of functional integration of radiology departments of more healthcare institutions; and,

• integrating medical imaging with the concept of an electronic patient record.

Deep theoretical background of PACS principle and into basic protocol DICOM is discussed in [1] and [2]. Brief technical introduction to the PACS system architecture is in [4,6,8].

Utilization of computer based medicine image processing brings new capabilities to the healthcare. Picture data can be processed and evaluated remotely in a reasonable time now. This approach allows to quickly ask for opinion of top specialists in case of a rare diseases diagnostics and ask for a second opinion or second reading in case where the radiologist is unsure.

1.2. MeDiMed project

Today most hospitals are using local PACS system serving only to one hospital. The goal of the MEDIMED project [7,10,11] is to initialize collaboration among hospitals as far as archiving and use of medical multimedia data and to provide the necessary technological infrastructure.

The Shared Regional PACS project MeDiMed started as a collaborative effort among Brno hospitals to process medical multimedia data. Masaryk University is the coordinator of this project ensuring that the demands and requirements of radiology departments are met, overseeing the changing legislative standards and the practical limitations of technology. Masaryk University, in cooperation with CESNET Association, also provides the necessary networking infrastructure.

Additionally, the project is to create conditions for general access to medical imaging data. The data exists already but its use is limited both in scope and time. By better utilization of the already existing equipment the project will bring a new quality into the healthcare operative, medical education and medical research as well as the decision-making on the level of local authorities.

The system deals with transmitting, archiving, and sharing medical image data originating from various medical modalities (computer tomography, magnetic resonance, ultrasound, mammography, etc.) from hospitals in the Brno metropolitan area. The Central PACS serves as a metropolitan communications node as well as a long term archive of patient's image studies.

Rather than creating just a computer network, it builds a network of medical specialists. This work not only impacts the healthcare field but also the education of medical specialists. The data stored in the shared archive can be made anonymous (i.e. personal data of patients is replaced by fictious data) and used for educational purposes.

Moreover, the process of making the data anonymous can be done in such a way that the data on a real patient obtained from several hospitals uses the same anonymous identity. That offers the students a more complex view of the evolution of the patient's health.

The realization of the project facilitates fast communication among individual hospitals, allows decision consultations, and brings various other advantages due to direct connections via optic networks. In general the MediMed project is clearly designed to support society-wide healthcare programs in the Czech Republic as well as programs implemented by other countries. The system is also supposed to serve as a learning tool for medical students of the Masaryk University as well as physicians in hospitals.

The gradual development of the joint system for processing and archiving image information is a natural step towards an increasing health care standard in the city of Brno and the whole region. Information on a patient's treatment in his own healthcare center as well as in other centers would be available. Consultations by more specialists will be enabled over the patent's picture, in case that a required specialist is not available in the center in question. Image information evaluation can be carried out in another place, general practitioners in the country will be able to consult specialists in hospitals, etc. Examination results will be available for the doctors in much shorter time than before. The implementation of the project has increased the speed of communication among individual hospitals, allowed decision consultations, and brought various other advantages due to dedicated network connections.

The realization of the project facilitates fast communication among individual hospitals, allows decision consultations, and brings various other advantages due to direct connections via optic networks. In general, the MeDiMed project is clearly designed to support common healthcare programs in the Czech Republic as well as programs implemented by other countries. The system is also supposed to serve as a learning tool for medical students of the Masaryk University as well as physicians in hospitals.

More detailed description of regional PACS system MeDiMEd and it step-by-step development is available in [4-6,8,12-14].

2. Technology used in MeDiMed

Medical picture data like X-Ray, CT, US, MR, etc. cannot be used without additional information like picture data description or evaluation, diagnosis, possibly a reference to the history of a patient's health, previous treatments and other information relevant to the patient. This complex set of information about a patient represents a very sensitive data.

Therefore high level of security for medical image data maintained by the regional PACS archive has to be provided. We have to secure the data in three stages: data stored on servers of the regional PACS, data transported over the network between this archive and the user, and users' access to these data.

The security of the data stored on the regional PACS servers is achieved by using dedicated hardware for this application and by strict limitation of the access (both physical and network based) to this equipment.

The security of the data transported over the network is provided by using dedicated fibre optics lines when available and by employing strong cryptography (IPSEC with AES-256 encryption algorithm) on all lines which are shared with other data traffic.

The main principle of the hospital-to-MeDiMed connection is the use of two firewalls. One of them is in front of the MeDiMed PACS servers and is under the control of the MeDiMed staff. The second one is the hospital's firewall and is controlled by the hospital staff. It allows us, as administrators of the application, to control the access to central resources and allows the administrators of the hospital's network to control the access to the hospital's network. That way all participants have the access to the network they are responsible for under their control. This principle applies to all types of connections (dedicated fiber optics or IPSEC tunnel) between the MeDiMed servers and the hospital. The structure is easy to see from Figure 2.

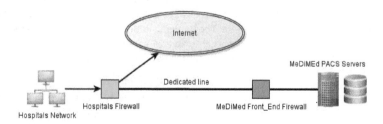

Figure 2. Common principle of the hospital to MeDiMed connection. There are two firewalls on the path form modalities and viewing stations to the PACS server. One of them is controlled by hospital and the second on by university.

Image distribution by specially configured dedicated computer networks plays a key role in the implementation of telemedicine. Every particular component of the whole system is certified so it can be integrated into the hospital information system infrastructure of cooperating healthcare institutions. All software tools are strictly based on the DICOM standard and could be easily incorporated into the already running systems.

The technology and networking solutions used in MeDiMed will be described in the following chapters.

2.1. Connections based on dedicated fibre optics

There is a large fibre optic cable network owned and operated by the universities in the city of Brno. The development of this network started in 1993. The ownership of the physical communication infrastructure is the key point for development and deployment of advanced networking services. MeDiMed is a good example of such a service.

The network is based on a fiber optic cable. Both, terrestrial and above ground, types of cable are used. The optical lines mostly have a ring topology for better reliability. This network interconnects all universities in the city and their faculties spread around whole city, various institutes of the Academy of Science, local government, courts, mostly all hospitals and some other institutions which were "on the road". Currently the network consists of about 150 km of optical cables and more than 90 nodes are using it.

The ownership of the private fiber optic network with enough free optics is mandatory for the implementation of new applications. It offers the freedom to establish private connections dedicated to these applications.

The development of computer networks is very fast as far as both the technology and the needs of network users are concerned. Since the beginnings of the Internet, full of enthusiasm of users and their happiness when the network was running at least sometimes we have moved through decades of manifold bandwidth raising (64 kbps was considered very good 15 years ago, today 100 Mbps is considered substandard) up to current state when a high performance internet connectivity is a standard. The users' demand for reliability has grown at a similar ratio.

In the beginning of the development of our network we used 10 Mbps Ethernet, mostly on a multimode fiber. At that time it was an economically acceptable solution corresponding with the level of technology of that time. In 1995 we started to use ATM because of the need for more bandwidth as well as the need for a dedicated transport channel for special applications. Today ATM is outdated in the area of data communication. However, at the time when FDDI was no longer a perspective technology and Fast Ethernet was not yet standardized, it was a reasonable solution. Both Ethernet and ATM network were built as a common open network of Masaryk University, Brno University of Technology and other academic parties. The ATM technology was the first one offering enough bandwidth and enough privacy to be able to support medicine multimedia data transport.

After the ATM age the networking technology moved to gigabit and ten-gigabit ethernet. This technology offers enough bandwidth and necessary services for a reasonable price. The second main change is the concept of an interconnection of the various institutions inside the metro-politan network. Terms like firewall and network security were not very common in the beginning of the Internet. Mail relays were open for everybody etc. At that time individual nodes of the metropolitan network were interconnected without any regard for the adminis-trative structure. The main criterion was technical and economical availability. With the development of the Internet, the principles of solidarity and academic cooperation have gradually been ignored. The Internet has become an everyday part of our lives and not everybody respects the privacy of the participating institutions. Contemporary networks are built in such a way that every institution makes a compact unit ensuring security from unwanted activity of other Internet users.

The application of medical multimedia data transport was constructed as an isolated and closed network. Only two hospitals with only one type of modality (ultrasound) were interconnected in the first stage via the ATM network. This interconnection was created as an ATM LANE network and a private IP address space was used. Step by step, more hospitals and more types of modalities have been connected. As far as technology is concerned, we have moved from ATM LANE to the private Fast Ethernet based on dedicated fiber optic pairs. A necessary prerequisite for this was the development of private fiber optic network. A dedicated fibre optics line can be dedicated to demanding applications as the private fibre optics cables contain enough free lines.

2.2. Encrypted tunnels

For hospitals along the scope of our fiber optics network we need to use dedicated lines leased from anybody who can offer it (very expensive solution) or public data network. The use of the public data network is more economical but it enforces utilization of strong cryptography for securing the data. IPSEC with AES-256 encryption algorithm is used for this purpose. The basic principle is kept as depicted on Figure 2. Typical interconnection of his type is on Figure 3.

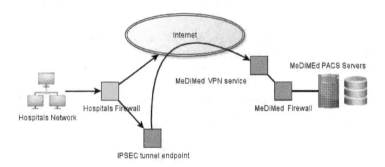

Figure 3. Connecting the hospital via IPSEC tunnel

2.3. Alien wavelength across the cesnet DWDM network

CESNET is an association originated by universities and Academy of science of Czech republic in 1996. Its main goal is to operate and develop academic backbone network of Czech republic. This network has started on lines with bandwidth in hundreds of kbps and step by step has grown to current backbone based on combination of ten-gigabit ethernet an even hundred gigabit etherent. The target speed of the core backbone is 100Gbps for the upcomming two years. The CESNET backbone interconnected all academic cities in republic.

CESNET provides services to education and research community. For research projects the budget is usually limited and the demand for special networks services (high bandwidth, low latency, certain level of privacy etc.) is very high. CESNET is a member of European research organisations like GEANT and is participating in a lot of research project in computer networks.

The CESNET backbone network is based on leased dark fiber lines enlighted by CESNET equipment. This is so called Custommer Empowered Fiber (CEF) approach. Dark fibre provides a lot of advantages and CESNET is using this technology on all backbone lines. DWDM technology is used in the core of the network. DWDM is used to provide data channels going through several backbone nodes. The real length of data channel may be several hundreds of kilometres. More detailed description of the CESNET backbone networks and technology solutions used to operate it is described in [16 – 19].

DWDM transport networks is traditionally used by service providers to offer clear channel services to its customers. Customers signal is typically carried as "gray" signal from customer's equipment to provider's equipment. This signal is inside transponder converted into "coloured" one and transported across DWDM providers network.

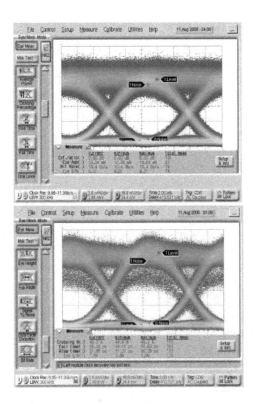

Figure 4. The eye diagram of signal used for testing of DWDM connection for Faculty Thoamyers' Hospital. The signal on the upper figure is clear signal generated by ten-gigabit ethernet pluggable module. The bottom figure is the weakest yet fully usable signal. Pictures are taken from [19].

Price of transponder is a mandatory part of the overall cost of DWDM service we've tried to use DWDM gigabit ethernet pluggable modules instead. The cost of these DWDM pluggables is several times lower than the price of corresponding transponder. The transponder provides more than just "colouring" of customers signal. It also ensures proper signal power. The length of the fiber line from transponder to the DWDM multiplex itself is usually few tens of centimetres. In case of utilisation of "coloured" custommers' signal the length of corresponding fiber span is typically several kilometres or tens of kilometres. The fiber optics line between customer and provider will introduce some attenuation of the signal. We have performed a set of lab measurements to learn the minimal input signal level of customer's DWDM signal that can ensure enough OSNR and guarantied BER. The eye diagrams from these testing are presented on Figure 4 just for better overview.

The first application of alien wavelength technology in CESNET was connection of Faculty Thomayers hospital in Prague to the MeDiMed PACS archive in Brno.

2.4. Wireless and satelite connections

As already mentioned, the backbone system uses optical wires as a transport medium. Nevertheless, only the hospitals in the city and several of the others in the republic are connected by optical wires.

Another transport medium which is being used is the radio connection. It may be utilized for the main connection of the locality, however in that case the bigger hospitals require at least 20-30 Mbit/s speed. We are speaking mainly about sending and storing pictures from MR, CT, and similar modalities where there is a high demand for transport capacity.

Fixed wireless connection is often used as the first mile of the hospital's connection to the public data network. We have optical connections between cities, but the fixed wireless connection is needed to connect the hospitals inside the city. This concerns establishing traffic in the paid band.

One of the biggest groups of the users of the wireless networks are the radiologists. They very frequently use the opportunity to create the descriptions of the pictures at home. That way, they may react to urgent cases immediately. There is no need to go to hospital and start working on a pressing case after a significant delay. Simultaneously, they save their time, because the work on the picture may often take significantly less of it, than the voyage.

Another technology, which we use for the MediMed project, is the satellite. Within the scope of HEALTHWARE project (which is a 6th EU framework program project), there are being installed terminal satellite devices to the places, where any proper connections are not existent. Some facilities, such as medical institutions for patients with tuberculosis, may be found in woodlands, areas without industrial burden. Than, the usage of a satellite system is one of the few ways, we may use for transfer of a medical information. It is therefore used despite its limited data capacity, that is so needed in the cases of urgent demands for transfer and processing of medical image data.

2.5. Mobile users

By scaling PACS outside of single hospital we meet with some limitations of DICOM protocol. DICOM was designed to be used inside one hospital. Inside one hospital where everything is under one common administration there is not necessary to have strong authentication mechanism. DICOM can identify its users only by IP address of the user's viewing station. In collaborative environment spread across more hospitals it may happen that the given medicine specialist needs to use more than one viewing station and vice versa the given viewing station is used by more specialists. Every medicine specialist should have access to different collections of patients picture data.

PACS users authentication in heterogenous environment (like regional PACS archive is) it is rather complicated. Lets recall most common cases of PACS usage.

First kind of PACS users are medicine modalities (X-Rays, CT, MR, etc.). Modalities are producing medicine picture data and storing it into PACS archive. Modalities have got a fixed IP address and a limited set of communication and authentication capabilities. From computer

science or networking point of view modalities are particular devices witch special communication requirements and should be served with respect to their natural properties. These
devices may be used by authorised personell only and security of data provided by these
equipments is guarantied by restricting physical access to these devices for authorised staff
only.

Dedicated viewing stations are special working places which serve for evaluation of picture
data obtained from modalities. This evaluation is performed by radiologiests or another
medicine specialists who are trained and sklilled specially for evaluation of medicine picture
data. These specialists should have access to all images obtained from modalities because they
are responsible for picture data interpretaion. Picture data description provided by radiologiests is in next step used by other medicine specialists for diagnosis assesment and treatment
of patient. Radiologists need a specialised hardware for proper work. From computer perspective this hardware can be identified by its IP address. This type of identification is sufficient
to authorise radiologist access to given medicine picture.

Physicians - experts in various branches of medicine - represent the most complicated part of
PACS users. Given physician should have access only to data concerning his patients,
sometimes patients of his department and in some special cases given patients of other
physicians. By special cases we mean first of all consultations asked by personal physician of
given patient. Physicians typically can access the PACS system from more than one computer
(from working place, from home or some times from other department of hospital). On the
other hand given computer may be shared by several physicians especially in case of specialised stations with graphics capabilities customised for viewing images from X-ray or other
particular modality. For this group of PACS users we have to provide proper authentication
mechanism.

The only authentication mechanism common to all used versions of DICOM is the IP address.
In case of modalities and viewing stations used by radiology deparment for medicine pictures
evaluation this is appropriate solution. We decided to use IP addresses also for authentication
of all other PACS users. Of course general IP address of workstation cannot be used as an user
identity. Pretty good solution seems to be utilisation of some properties of IPSEC.

In this case the user is authenticated by his publis RSA key. After successfull authentication
an IPSEC tunnel is established between users workstation and dedicated IPSEC server used
by regional PACS. IPSEC server then assignes tunnel IP address to the user's station. User
authentication in the PACS system is then based on the tunnel IP address.

PACS users identity is based on PKI infrastructure. Each user who needs to use more than one
station or who is sharing viewing staions with others will be provided by an USB dongle
containing his private RSA key. The key is generated on the dongle and never leaves it. So it's
really very difficult for anybody else then the authorised user to use it. The corresponding
public key is signed by regional PACS certification authority. A dedicated certification
authority is used at this moment. The problem of electronic identity of physicians should be
solved globally for the whole healthcase system in the future.

2.6. Redundancy

The key services of the regional PACS system are running in two distinct locations. The MeDiMed services can provide better reliability and availability this way. MeDiMed is able to survive the failure of any single fibre optics line, server, storage, electricity (though it is backed up via UPS and motor-generator) in one location and even a failure of the PACS system software in one location. The global view on this system is illustrated on Figure 5.

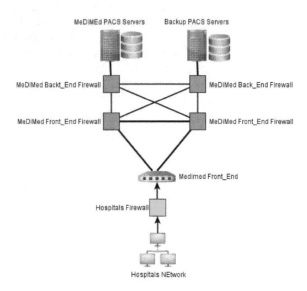

Figure 5. Detail of MeDiMed redundant infrastructure.

Networking infrastructure offers redundant connectivity for both local and remote hospitals. For local hospitals there are two independent fibre optics lines. One line connects the hospital to the primary location and the second one to the backup location. Remote hospitals utilize IPSEC tunnels also connected to both locations. The critical single point of fail for them is the connection to public data network. This connection is usually unprotected.

The MeDiMed project utilises a lot of servers for many different applications. For all applications provided to the MeDiMed users we have to offer a reliable enough service.

There is a set of PACS servers used for a routine storage of medical images. The PACS server for this type of service runs on a dedicated hardware in both university sites used by MeDiMed. Primary and backup PACS servers servicing the given hospital or providing given particular service work as two standalone and mostly independend servers. Data from the primary server are replicated to the backup one via DICOM protocol. One site is a primary site and, until it fails, all images are stored on this location. The second site serves as a backup location and all data are automatically copied from the master servers to the backup servers. The backup servers are available at all times for retrieving of medical images in the read-only mode. This way the overall performance of the system can be improved. If the master site fails we can manually switch the backup site to the read-write mode and the former master site to the read-only mode. In many cases the primary and the backup PACS servers are from different vendors. Even though, bidirectional synchronisation of the PACS servers is more complicated in this case. The manual switching of primary and backup PACS servers provides good enough service with regards to the number of failures. Moreover, modalities have some local cache so that they can keep images for several days. Older images are available for reading on both primary and backup sites.

Another large set of PACS servers are so called communication PACS servers. That means PACS servers used for an interchange of medical images between healthcare institutions. Unlike the PACS servers used for routine storage of medical images, the communication PACS servers have to be switched automatically. Communication PACS retrieves the image from one client and offers it to another one. Clients have to manually switch to backup communication PACS server in case of failure of the primary one.

We have considered a cluster of two hardware servers, preferably located in two different sites of the network. Even though this solution seems to be popular, well known and tested, it is not suitable for PACS servers used in MeDiMed. The utilisation of hardware clusters needs some basic support from applications. Hardware failure may occur at any time and any stage of data processing, especially at any stage of storing the data into the database or simply writing the data into the disk subsystem. The time granularity of copying the raw image from a master to a slave system more or less corresponds to the heartbeat frequency. In the case of the master to slave switching we may lose data processed since the last heartbeat tick to the failure of the master system. The application should assume such situation and enclose the critical operations into transactions to allow recovery from the master hardware failure. Most communication PACS servers used in MeDiMed do not expect to run in a cluster environment.

2.7. InstantPACS system

Small healthcare institutions and private doctor's offices are being more and more equipped with diagnostics devices like CT X-ray ultrasound etc. The small healthcare institutions demand for medicine picture data processing capabilities and services is coming right now. MeDiMed intends to offer PACS services also to these new perspective medicine users. The specific property of PACS or any ICT services in small healthcare institution is lack of technical staff capable to solve issues on place. For this reason we are developing an "all-in-one" device which will serve as local PACS server for the healthcare institution and provide backup and communication services. Development and deployment of such a system is coved by the InstantPACS project.

The aim of the InstantPACS project is to develop a maintenance-free PACS system suitable for small and midsized healthcare institutions. This PACS system will offer to the small healthcare institutions a user amenity obvious in hospitals including e.g. automatic backup of medicine data. The most important properties of this system are user friendliness, maintenance free operations and pricing acceptable for private doctor's offices. The InstantPACS project is an integral part of the MeDiMed shared regional PACS server overlay project.

InstantPACS is remotely controllable and from point of view of users is not asking for any local maintenance. General user of the InstantPACS will be private doctor's office. A private doctor's office is typically equipped with an ultrasound and one or two more modalities like CT. Modalities in private doctor's office are from point of view of data communication isolated devices. Data from these modalities are usually transported on a USB sticks or processed locally on the modality's console. It is necessary to interconnect modalities and viewing stations in the doctor's office to offer medical picture processing comfort usual in large hospitals. Once the data will be transported from the modality outside it is necessary to provide at least the following services:

- transport data to the viewing station

- backup the data to an external device or PACS system

- long term archive of the data

- prevent any unauthorized access to the data

- allow to share data between authorized users

The InstantPACS server is used in a very similar manner like PACS systems in large hospitals. Of course there are some technology discrepancies given by different server placement possibilities in large hospitals (dedicated computer room with air conditioning enough space etc.) and private doctor's offices (one room shared by treatments and server hosting, room temperature etc). These worst environmental conditions have introduced some Instant-PACS server hardening demands. Backup of medicine picture data from Instant PACS server will be performed on two backup PACS servers located at Masaryk University. The data communication will be performed over Internet via two tunnels protected by strong cryptography used as shown on Figure 6.

The key requirement is no or as small as possible regular local maintenance of the system. Users of the InstantPACS are expected to have no or very little experience with management of servers operating systems etc. On the other hand we expect rather large number of users. All critical events and states should be automatically detected and reported. Also some extensions of the installed system like addition of new modality (which is typically performed by trained ICT staff in large hospitals) should be solvable in an intuitive way.

The hardware platform used for InstantPACS is based on off-the-shelf components and was tailored especially to this project. It has dedicated memory for system software and configuration and redundant disk subsystem for storage of medicine picture data. It can contain embedded ethernet switch to connect few modalities in a typical private doctor's office. IPSEC tunnels for backup data encryption are terminated directly in the InstantPACS so no additional equipment is needed.

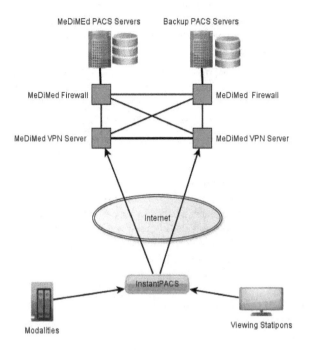

Figure 6. Common principle of InstantPACS communication with the centralized PACS servers.

2.8. Monitoring

The amount of various equipments used in MeDiMed is increasing during MeDiMed development and new functionalities deployment. The amount of used equipment and the increasind demand for reliability and availability of MeDiMed services enforced development of centralised monitoring system. This monitoring system provides all the necessary supplemental services like collecting of traffic statistics, networking devices configuration backup, time synchronisation, network administrators authentication, etc.

Two Linux based servers are used as central management stations. These servers are working independently and are located at both of the MeDiMed centrall locations. The primary management station is located at the Institute of Computer Science of Masaryk University and the second one is located at the Faculty of Medicine. Each management station provides full set of services. Monitoring servers form a redundant solution for all the goals listed above.

Both of the monitoring servers are running Nagios. Nagios is a popular open source software platform. It is widely used to network component status, servers CPU utilisation and number of running processes, disk storage utilization and many others.

The whole monitoring system is accessible via web interface and provides the current status as well as the history of all equipments and services availability. Critical alarms are propagated via SMS messages distributed via SMS Siemens 35i terminals directly connected over RS232 interface to both management servers.

The monitoring servers are collecting syslog messages as well. Syslog messages are parsed and processed on daily basis. The resulting file provides both statistics of stored medical image studies, DICOM pictures provided by separate modalities and errors encountered by all PACS servers. This summary result is distributed via e-mail daily.

It is very useful to have remote access to console interfaces of both servers and networking devices especially for emergency cases. A set of KVM (Keyboard-Video-Mouse) switches are used in both primary and backup locations for this purpose. KVM switches offer remote access via web interface. Dedicated Cisco routers are used to connect those KVM switches to the data network. These routers also provide access to console interfaces of networking equipment via reverse telnet. Access to KVM switches and other console ports from outside of the dedicated MEDiMEd wolrd is permitted only via IPSEC tunnels ended directly on the above mentioned routers. This approach provides us emergency secure access to management interfaces of all key equipments.

3. Benefit of cooperation in medicine

Many PACS installations are only limited to the scope of a particular radiology department or work as a repository of a single modality. An effective usage of that technology means image distribution at least throughout the whole healthcare institution. However, the most promising approach for exploiting of PACS technology is to use it at the regional or national level and to support the associated medical processes that way.

By effective usage is meant not only basic support of daily routines in radiology departments but also the support of distant consultations, digital long-term archiving and development of shared knowledge databases for research and education.

MeDiMed project brings a new quality into healthcare, medical education and medical research as well as the treatment decision-making.

3.1. Cooperation on the area of medicine picture data processing

The is a set of so called communications PACS servers inside the MeDiMed. Communication PACS server means PACS server used for interchange of medicine images between healthcare institutions. Communications PACS subsystem allows medicine specialist to share the picture data for diagnosis consultations second reading or even load balancing of radiologists.

The MeDiMed platform supports the cooperation it the area of processing of medical image information also in international scale. For example the Healthware (Standard and interoperable satellite solution to deploy health care services over wide areas) project within the sixth framework programme of EU covers many telemedicine activities.

The goal of the Healthware project is developing of healthcare services over the satellite network to increase quality and comfort in European medical practices. The aim is to bridge the medical digital divide in Europe by designing, integrating and validating interoperable telecoms and services platforms to provide existing and future healthcare services. The satellite based platforms can interact with mobile and terrestrial technologies to supply effective and reliable end-to-end healthcare services and boost the deployment of large-scale satellite communications telemedicine services.

Additionally, Healthware will have a beneficial effect on training and education as far as 7 Universities and Research Centres are concerned. For undergraduate, post-graduate and PhD students, the participation in such programs is a unique opportunity to be exposed to team work with regular reporting and evaluation by the partners. The research performed is usually of very high quality due to the number experts involved in the group and the concentration of financial resources. It is also the occasion to be exposed to a multicultural environment and to establish international relationships that are very useful to build and strengthen the European Research Area.

3.2. Medical training support

Teaching has always been one of the most important parts of radiology. The fundamental principle is very simple. Every radiology department participating in teaching of medical students or in research is equipped with specialized diagnostic workstation. This workstation must be primarily connected to their hospital PACS system or other equipment generating image studies in DICOM format.

Images appropriate for teaching and research purposes are made anonymous (i.e. the personal data of the patient and other information that may disclose the patient's identity is replaced by fictitious information) when sending into Educational and Research PACS. One of the basic principles when sending images into the Educational and Research PACS is the coordinated assignment of fictitious patient identity, so it can offer a more complex view of the evolution of the patients health in situations where the patient is being treated in different healthcare facilities. Therefore, the legal barrier preventing access to sensitive and confidential patient data is removed.

The database of anonymized CT images is populated by senior medicine specialists. It is used by medicine students and by novice medicine doctors as well.

The education superstructure consists of Case Study objects. Every Case Study object is hypertext document describing given medical case and referencing relevant anonymized medical image studies. Case Study is accessible via standard www browser and if there is specialized diagnostic viewer installed on this computer then referenced image can be manipulated and processed appropriate way using all possibilities supported by particular viewer. It means that students of medical faculties could access huge amount of interesting systematized medical image information related to their subject from their teaching rooms. Teaching room equipped with appropriate software can also serve as trainer for young radiologists. This way they can learn new technologies, compare hardware and software of different diagnostic workstations.

The core of our solution is tailored PACS. That PACS can be used as a "PACS trainer" for students and young radiologists but also forms the basis for additional educational and research applications such as for example the Case Studies describing treatment of real patients. The Case Study is an integrated hypertext document forming didactic unit and consists of short texts, structured clinical data, radiological images of various kinds, images from nuclear medicine modalities, macroscopic and microscopic pathology images or demonstration of the video movies recorded during surgeries.

The Case Study can be accessible via standard web browser and if the users have DICOM diagnostic workstation installed on their computers, then the referenced image study can be manipulated and processed in all ways supported by the particular workstation. It means that medical students can access large amounts of systematized medical cases related to their subject. The labs equipped with appropriate software can also serve as training simulators for those training to be radiologists. The students can learn more practical lessons instead of wasting their time in the library.

Every image study must be annotated with a detailed description in DICOM Structured Report format and every image must also be assigned a set of key words describing all the medical findings and diagnosis for better retrieval of specific cases. Data on the real patient obtained from several hospitals uses the same fictitious identity, thereby offering students a more complex view of the evolution of the patient's health.

Educational and Research PACS solution also supports utilization of sets of key words making a search for specific image studies easier. An automatic evaluation of answers regarding prepared collections of images that are not described, used for medical students' examination purposes, etc. and provide an additional benefit.

4. Conclusion

The MeDiMed project has started a deeper collaboration among hospitals in the area of processing of medical multimedia data and to provide the necessary technological infrastructure for this cooperation. Additionally, the project created conditions for general access to medical imaging data.

The implementation of the MeDiMed project facilitates fast communication among individual hospitals, allows decision consultations, and offers capabilities of today's computer systems and data networks to medical users. Moreover, the system is supposed to serve as a learning tool for medical students as well as physicians in hospitals participating in this project.

The gradual development of the joint system for processing and archiving image information is a positive step towards increasing the healthcare standard in the city of Brno as well as in the whole region.

Information on a patient's treatment in his/her own healthcare center as well as in other centers would be available, review and consultations regarding the patient's data by more specialists will be enabled, image information evaluation can be carried out in another place in case a required specialist is not available in the center in question, general practitioners in the country will be able to consult specialists in hospitals, etc. Examination results will be available for the doctors in much shorter time than before.

The development of the system for processing, archiving and accessing the patients' image information, designed in this way, contributes to a significant improvement of the patients' image information and to significant improvement of the patients' care. It enables consultation with specialists not only within a region but also outside the country. Created data files enable practitioners to carry out evaluation of the treatment as well as administered medication in a large sample of patients.

The new goal for the MeDiMed project is to offer PACS system to small institutions. Small healthcare institutions and private doctor's offices usually have limited data network availability. They are typically located near patients and data communication is not they priority. ICT staff in such institutions is also very limited if it exists at all. For this reason the solution used by large hospitals is not suitable for small institutions. Even though the basic principles used in large hospitals can be preserved also in this case.

Current ICT, as well as existing and developing standards, enable physicians to deliver some services through the computer network. It means that medical specialists from distant specialized departments can consult urgent cases or make decisions. It is a concept of expert centers based on the practices of telemedicine. Image studies of every patient can be referred to a distant expert center for a primary diagnostic or second opinion. This way a much higher quality diagnosis can be assured.

Another important application of the shared regional PACS servers is education. Interesting cases are anonymized and used for both education and research. The shared regional collaborative environment is more than just a set of computer network applications. Gradually, it changes the thinking of medical specialists and enables them to cooperate and share data about patients in electronic form. It builds a network of medical specialists. The implementation of the system has increased the speed of communication among individual hospitals, allowed decision consultations, and brought various other advantages due to dedicated network connections.

Author details

Karel Slavicek, Michal Javornik and Otto Dostal

Institute of Computer Science Masaryk University, Czech Republic

References

[1] Dreyer D. K., Hirschorn J. S., Thrall A., Mehta H., PACS A Guide to the Digital Revolution, 2006, Springer Science +Business Media, Inc., USA, ISBN 978-0387-26010-5

[2] H. K. Huang, DSc, PACS and Imaging Informatics: Basic Principles and Applications, Hoboken, NJ: Wiley, 2004 ISBN 0-471-25123-2.

[3] DICOM 3.0 Standard. [Online]. Available: http://www.nema.org/stds/2007-DICOM-FULLSET.cfm.

[4] Petrenko M., Ventruba P., Dostal O., First application of Picture Archiving and Communication System (PACS) in Gynecologic Endoscopy, ISGE - 6th Regional Meeting, Bangkog. ISGE 2002, 53-56

[5] Dostal O., Filka M., Petrenko M., University computer network and its application for multimedia transmissin in medicine, WSEAS Int. Conf. on Information Security, Harware/Software Codesign, E-Commerce and Computer Networks, Rio de Janeiro, Brasil. WSEAS 2002, 1961-1964

[6] Petrenko M., Dostal O., Ventruba P., First Experiences with Picture Archiving and Communication Systems (PACS) in gynecology, Israel Journal of Obstetrics and Gynecology, 2001, vol. 2000, no. 3, 128-130

[7] Dostal O., Javornik M., Petrenko M., Slavicek K., MEDIMED-Regional Centre for Archiving and Interhospital Exchange of Medicine Multimedia Data. In Proceedings of the Second IASTED International Conference on Communications, Internet, and Information Technology. Scottsdale, Arizona, USA : International Association of Science and Technology for Development- IASTED, 2003. ISBN 0-88986-398-9, s. 609-614. 2003, Scottsdale Arizona USA

[8] Dostal O., Filka M., Petrenko M., New Possibilities of Multimedia Applications in Medicine, Proceeeding of ELMAR-2004, 46-th International Symposium Electonics in Marine, 16-18 June 2004, Zadar Croatia, ISSN 1334-2630, p. 402-405

[9] Dostal O., Filka M., Slavicek K., Videoconference using ATM in medicine. In Telecommunications and Signal Processing TSP 99. Brno : FEI VUT BRNO, 1999. ISBN 80-214-4154-6, s. 195-3 s. 1999, Brno.

[10] Dostal O., Javornik M., Slavicek K., Petrenko M., Andres P., Development of Regional Centre for Medical Multimedia Data Processing, Proceedings of the Third IASTED International Conferee on Communications, Internet and Information Technology. St.Thomas, US Virgin Islands: International Association of Science and Technology for Development- IASTED, 2004. ISBN 0-88986-445-4, p.632-636.

[11] Schmidt M., Dostal O., Javornik M., MEDIMED - Regional PACS Centre in Brno, Czech Republic, Proceedings of the 22th International Conference of EuroPACS& MIR (Managenment in Radiology) Conference, 16 - 18 September, Trieste, Italy

[12] Dostal O., Javornik M., Regional Educational and Research Centre for Processing of Medical Image Information, CARS 2005 Computer Assisted Radiology and Surgery, June 22.-25. 2005, Berlin, Germany, p.911-915. ISBN 0-444-51872-X, ISSN 0531-5131.

[13] Dostal O., Javornik M., Ventruba P., Collaborative environment supporting research and education in the area of medical image information. International Journal of Computer Assisted Radiology and Surgery, Deutschland : Springer, ISSN 1861-6410, 2006, pp. 98-100,

[14] Dostal O., Javornik M., Slavicek K., Opportunity of Current ICT in the Processing of Medical Image Information. In IASTED International Conference on Advances in Computer Science and Technology. Puerto Vallarta, Mexico, S. Sahni, Ed. IASTED/ ACTA Press, 2006, pp. 193–195.

[15] Dostal O., Slavicek K., Wireless Technology in Medicine Applications. In PWC, ser. IFIP, R. Bestak, B. Simak, and E. Kozlowska, Eds., vol. 245. Springer, 2007, pp. 316– 324.

[16] Altmanova L., Sima S., Towards a Nation-wide Fibre Footprint in Research and Education Networking. Rhodes, TERENA, 9. 6. 2004, Rhodes

[17] Novak V., Slavicek K., Cihlar J., Forghieri A., Design and Deployment of CESNET2 DWDM Core Network, in CESNET Conference 2006, CESNET, z. s. p. o., 2006, str.: 43;53 , ISBN: 80-239-6533-6

[18] Slavicek K., Novak V., Cesnet Backbone Transport Network. WSEAS Transactions on Communications, vol. 6, no. 2, pp. 377–382, 2007.

[19] Slavicek K., Novak V., Introduction of Alien Wavelength into Cesnet DWDM Backbone. In Sixth International Conference on Information, Communications and Signal Processing. IEEE, 2007.

Permissions

The contributors of this book come from diverse backgrounds, making this book a truly international effort. This book will bring forth new frontiers with its revolutionizing research information and detailed analysis of the nascent developments around the world.

We would like to thank Dongqing Wang, for lending his expertise to make the book truly unique. He has played a crucial role in the development of this book. Without his invaluable contribution this book wouldn't have been possible. He has made vital efforts to compile up to date information on the varied aspects of this subject to make this book a valuable addition to the collection of many professionals and students.

This book was conceptualized with the vision of imparting up-to-date information and advanced data in this field. To ensure the same, a matchless editorial board was set up. Every individual on the board went through rigorous rounds of assessment to prove their worth. After which they invested a large part of their time researching and compiling the most relevant data for our readers. Conferences and sessions were held from time to time between the editorial board and the contributing authors to present the data in the most comprehensible form. The editorial team has worked tirelessly to provide valuable and valid information to help people across the globe.

Every chapter published in this book has been scrutinized by our experts. Their significance has been extensively debated. The topics covered herein carry significant findings which will fuel the growth of the discipline. They may even be implemented as practical applications or may be referred to as a beginning point for another development. Chapters in this book were first published by InTech; hereby published with permission under the Creative Commons Attribution License or equivalent.

The editorial board has been involved in producing this book since its inception. They have spent rigorous hours researching and exploring the diverse topics which have resulted in the successful publishing of this book. They have passed on their knowledge of decades through this book. To expedite this challenging task, the publisher supported the team at every step. A small team of assistant editors was also appointed to further simplify the editing procedure and attain best results for the readers.

Our editorial team has been hand-picked from every corner of the world. Their multi-ethnicity adds dynamic inputs to the discussions which result in innovative outcomes. These outcomes are then further discussed with the researchers and contributors who give their valuable feedback and opinion regarding the same. The feedback is then collaborated with the researches and they are edited in a comprehensive manner to aid the understanding of the subject.

Apart from the editorial board, the designing team has also invested a significant amount of their time in understanding the subject and creating the most relevant covers. They scrutinized every image to scout for the most suitable representation of the subject and create an appropriate cover for the book.

The publishing team has been involved in this book since its early stages. They were actively engaged in every process, be it collecting the data, connecting with the contributors or procuring relevant information. The team has been an ardent support to the editorial, designing and production team. Their endless efforts to recruit the best for this project, has resulted in the accomplishment of this book. They are a veteran in the field of academics and their pool of knowledge is as vast as their experience in printing. Their expertise and guidance has proved useful at every step. Their uncompromising quality standards have made this book an exceptional effort. Their encouragement from time to time has been an inspiration for everyone.

The publisher and the editorial board hope that this book will prove to be a valuable piece of knowledge for researchers, students, practitioners and scholars across the globe.

List of Contributors

Kristie M. Guite, J. Louis Hinshaw and Fred T. Lee Jr.
Department of Radiology, University of Wisconsin, Madison, WI, USA

Fathinul Fikri Ahmad Saad, Abdul Jalil Nordin and Hishar Hassan
Centre for Diagnostic Nuclear imaging, University Putra Malaysia, Serdang, Selangor, Malaysia

Cheah Yoke Kqueen
Biomedicine Unit Faculty of Medicine and Health Science, University Putra Malaysia, Serdang, Selangor, Malaysia

W.F.E Lau
Department of Radiology, the University of Melbourne, Centre for Molecular Imaging, The Peter MacCallum, Cancer Centre, Australia

Y.I. Sumita, H. Taniguchi and M. Hattori
Department of Maxillofacial Prosthetics, Graduate School, Tokyo Medical and Dental University, Japan

K. Inohara
Department of Maxillofacial Prosthetics, Graduate School, Tokyo Medical and Dental University, Japan
Keishu-kai Inohara Dental Clinic, Japan

R. Sakurai
Shinjuku-nishiguchi Dental Clinic, Japan

S. Ino
Human Technology Research Institute, National Institute of Advanced Industrial Science and Technology, Japan

T. Ifukube
Institute of Gerontology, The University of Tokyo, Japan

Karel Slavicek, Michal Javornik and Otto Dostal
Institute of Computer Science Masaryk University, Czech Republic